National Children's Bureau Bibliographies

2

The Child with Cerebral Palsy

Rosemary Dinnage

NFER-NELSON

618.92836

DIN

Published by The NFER-NELSON Publishing Company Ltd.,
Darville House, 2 Oxford Road East,
Windsor, Berkshire SL4 1DF, England

and in the United States of America by

NFER-NELSON, 242 Cherry Street, Philadelphia, PA 19106–1906.
Tel: (215) 238 0939. Telex: 244489.

First Published 1986
© 1986 National Children's Bureau

Library of Congress Cataloging in Publication data

Dinnage, Rosemary.
    The child with cerebral palsy.

    Updated version of: The child with cerebral palsy / Doris Pilling.
1973.
    Includes index.
    1. Cerebral palsy – Psychological aspects – Abstracts. 2. Cerebral
palsy – Social aspects – Abstracts. 3. Cerebral palsied children –
Rehabilitation – Abstracts. 4. Cerebral palsied children – Education
– Abstracts. I. Pilling, Doria. Child with cerebral palsy. II. Title.
RJ496.C4D56   1986   618.92'836   85–32093
ISBN 0–7005–1022–2

Photoset by David John (Services) Ltd., Maidenhead

Printed in Great Britain by Henry Ling Ltd., at the Dorset Press, Dorchester, Dorset

ISBN 0–7005–1022–2
Code 8208 02 1

23.6.97

This book is due for return on or before the last date shown below.

The C

Contents

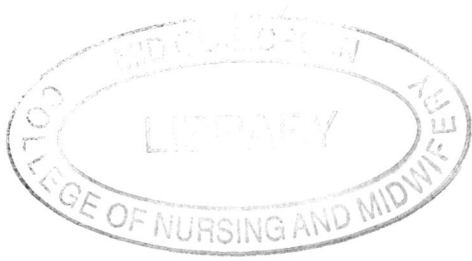

Acknowledgements

Thanks are due first to the Department of Health and Social Security whose grant made this review possible.

The National Children's Bureau librarians, Ian Vallender and Biddy Cunnell, provided invaluable help in searching for references and obtaining books and photocopies. The librarian of the Tavistock Centre, Margaret Walker, was most helpful in providing further references by means of a computer scan. The library of the Spastics Society was also made available to the author.

Thanks are due in particular to Professor Lewis Rosenbloom, who read the manuscript and made constructive suggestions. Finally, Doria Pilling, author of the booklets in their first edition, is not only responsible for part of the contents but has kindly advised on the updated version.

Introduction

In 1972–73 the National Children's Bureau published a series of concise research review booklets on childhood handicaps. Non-medical studies were summarized, and a brief overview added. In the years since, a great deal of further research and discussion has been published, and the Bureau felt it would be useful to have updated versions. The new booklets, therefore, contain material that was in the originals, together with more recent entries; and the reviews prefacing the annotated bibliographies have been rewritten.

The present booklet is concerned with research on children with cerebral palsy. Cerebral palsy is the term used to describe a group of non-progressive disorders occurring in young children in which impairment of motor function is caused by a lesion above the brain stem (Ingram *et al.*, 1964a, b and Rutter, Graham and Yule, 1970a, b (see Sections II and IV)). While all children with cerebral palsy have some difficulty in motor control, this difficulty takes a number of different forms, the extent of the handicap varies and there are considerable differences in severity. The brain damage causing the motor impairment may also cause a wide variety of additional handicaps – these include intellectual retardation, epilepsy, speech and hearing defects and visual, perceptual and visuo-motor impairments. Under the category of cerebral palsy then are children with a diversity of handicaps.

SECTION I
Attitudes to Cerebral Palsy

Although an extensive literature on attitudes to the disabled now exists, very few studies relate specifically to cerebral palsy. Most of those that deal directly with it have been primarily concerned with finding an order of preference for various types of disability, a rather artificial method of assessing attitudes (Shears and Jensema, 1969; Tringo, 1970). Findings – using samples of high school children, college students and adults – are unanimous that the cerebral palsied are seen by the non-handicapped – as a friend, co-worker, playmate for child, marriage partner – less favourably than those with sensory handicaps or physical handicaps without brain involvement. The cerebral palsied tend to be particularly stigmatized by the visibility of their handicap. Attitudes may vary in different countries; Sanua (1970) found more prejudice in the less industrialized countries.

One study (Combs and Harper, 1967) has assessed the effect of the 'label' cerebral palsy. Teachers and education students perceived a description of the behaviour of a handicapped child more favourably when it was presented to them unlabelled than when the label of cerebral palsy was attached.

There are a few studies of the cerebral palsied child's school life (listed in later sections) which suggest that in ordinary schools he or she is less popular than his or her classmates and may attract teasing (Marlow et al., 1968 and Anderson, 1973 (see Section IV); O'Moore, 1980; Anderson et al., 1982 (see Section II)). O'Moore and Anderson both found teachers in their samples to be not fully aware of the problem.

It would be wrong to conclude, though, that the non-handicapped simply have a negative attitude to the cerebral palsied. Research on general attitudes to the physically handicapped (summarized in the companion volume *The Orthopaedically Handicapped Child* (Dinnage, 1986)) has indicated that they are multi-dimensional, in some situations the handicapped being treated more favourably than the non-handicapped. As Altman (1981) points out, feelings about illness and disability are highly complex, and the research has often been simplistic. A point that emerges from several studies (Rapier et al., 1972; Donaldson and Martinson, 1977; Handlers and Austin, 1980; Rosenbaum and Armstrong, 1984) is that personal contact with the disabled has far more effect than theoretical instruction. Although prejudice affects early encounters, thereafter attitudes are modified by the personal characteristics of the handicapped person. In spite of these qualifications, however, it is clear that the cerebral palsied child does still have to face much fear, ignorance and prejudice.

1

BARSCH, R.H.
(1964)
*American Journal
of Public Health,*
54, 9, 1560–7.

The handicapped ranking scale among parents of handicapped children

2375 subjects, including nurses, professional therapists, teachers, students and parents of handicapped children, were asked to rank ten handicapping conditions (cerebral palsy, mental retardation, mental illness, brain injury, blindness, epilepsy, deafness, polio, heart trouble, diabetes) in the order of their severity for a child. There was wide agreement that cerebral palsy was the most severe handicap. Parents of cerebral palsied children saw some handicaps (mental retardation or mental illness) as more serious than their child's, but still ranked cerebral palsy high in severity.

COMBS, R.H. and
HARPER, J.L.
(1967)
*Exceptional
Children,* 33, 6,
399–403.

Effects of labels on attitudes of educators towards handicapped children

It has been suggested that adults may react to a handicapped child according to their attitudes to the term or 'label' used to describe the handicapping condition rather than to the child's actual behaviour. In this study 80 experienced teachers and 80 education students were found to perceive descriptions of the behaviour of four types of handicapped children differently when labels were attached than when the descriptions were presented unlabelled. The effect of labelling was not uniform, for while cerebral palsied, psychopathic and schizophrenic children were perceived more negatively when their descriptions were labelled, mentally retarded children were assessed more favourably when labelled. No differences in attitudes to the handicapped children were found between the teachers and the students.

SHEARS, L.M.
and JENSEMA,
C.J.
(1969)
*Exceptional
Children,* 36, 2,
91–6.

Social acceptability of anomalous persons

Ninety-four subjects (college students or attendants in state institutions for the mentally retarded) were asked to rank ten types of physically or mentally handicapped or socially deviant person according to their acceptability in various social situations. In most situations those with cerebral palsy were less acceptable than those with a visible disability (e.g. the amputee or blind) or a communication disorder (e.g. the deaf or a stutterer) but more acceptable than those whose condition was associated with stigma (the mentally ill, retarded or homosexual). When the cerebral palsied person was considered as a marriage partner, however, he or she joined the lowest group in acceptability. It is suggested that different factors underlie acceptability in different social situations.

SANUA, V.
(1970)
Social Science and Medicine, 4, 5, 461–512.

A cross cultural study of cerebral palsy

A pilot study designed to test the hypothesis that the degree of psychological adjustment of a cerebral palsied person is related to the socio-cultural values and economic structure of the society in which he or she lives. Subjects were 250 adolescents and young adults with cerebral palsy attending rehabilitation centres or vocational schools in eight European countries.

A battery of psychological tests was given to the subjects. In general, there was a tendency for more favourable attitudes to disability to be found in subjects from the more advanced countries, particularly England and northern France, and less favourable attitudes in those from the less industrialized countries, particularly Spain, Portugal and Israel (half of the Israeli subjects came from Moslem countries originally). An interesting finding was the high quality of stories from the French subjects (on the Thematic Apperception Test), which the author attributes to the emphasis placed on verbal and literary fluency in the French educational system. The study gives some indication of the importance of socio-cultural values. Further research, with more representative samples, is recommended.

TRINGO, J.L.
(1970)
Journal of Special Education, 4, 3, 295–306.

The hierarchy of preference towards disability groups

455 subjects from six sample groups, including high school and college students and rehabilitation workers, were asked to indicate the closest relationship they would allow to a person in each of 21 disability groups. A similar order of preference was found in all the sample groups. Generally the physically disabled were the most acceptable, then the sensory disabled, while the brain-injured were the least acceptable. Cerebral palsy was the eighth least acceptable disability, with the hunchback, tuberculosis, ex-convict, mental retardation, alcoholism and mental illness being less acceptable.

RAPIER, J.,
ADELSON, R.,
CAREY, R., and
CROKE, K.
(1972)
*Exceptional
Children*, 39, 3,
219–23.

Changes in children's attitudes towards the physically handicapped

From a school in California incorporating a unit for the orthopaedically handicapped, 152 children aged 8 to 11 were asked about their attitudes to the handicapped before and after a year of integrated schooling. Even before integration their attitudes were quite positive, but they changed in terms of seeing the handicapped children as not so weak and helpless as they had thought. Before integration there were sex differences in attitudes, but these disappeared after integration. Integrated schooling is valuable in changing children's negative stereotypes of handicap.

DONALDSON, J.
and MARTINSON,
M.C.
(1977)
*Exceptional
Children*, 43, 6,
337–41.

Modifying attitudes towards physically disabled persons

Subjects were 120 non-disabled university students of both sexes, assigned to four experimental groups. A discussion was held with six visibly handicapped young people (cerebral palsy, blindness, etc). One group of subjects sat in on a discussion with these people about their lives; one group saw a video of the discussion; one group heard a tape of it; one group did none of these things. All subjects filled in an 'Attitude Toward Disabled Persons Scale' afterwards. Results suggest that both a live and a videotaped discussion were effective in changing students' attitudes towards the disabled. There were no significant differences betwen male and female students' reactions. The use of such a videotape in education is discussed.

WEINBERG, N.
(1978)
*Rehabilitation
Counselling
Bulletin*, 21, 3,
183–9.

Preschool children's perceptions of orthopedic disability

Children of three, four and five were tested on their understanding of orthopaedic handicap. On the first experiment they were divided into two groups; half were shown a photograph of an able-bodied child and half of a child in a wheelchair. They were asked if they would like to play with the child, whether the child could run, sing, and colour, and whether teacher and parents would want them to play with the handicapped children. They were then asked questions to determine whether they understood the disability involved. It was clear that understanding increased dramatically after three years of age. No differences were found at any age on the questions about liking, parental approval, and the handicapped child's abilities.

On the second experiment another group of three- to five-year-olds were shown similar pictures and asked which of the two children they would rather play with. They were again asked questions to test their understanding of disability; and again, understanding seemed to come by four or five years. 73 per cent of the children preferred the able-bodied child as a playmate, the percentage rising with age. No sex differences were found in either experiment. The findings suggest that the attitudes of young children are flexible, as they only showed preference for the able-bodied when specifically asked to choose. Education about disability should evidently be started early.

HANDLERS, A.
and AUSTIN, K.
(1980)
*Exceptional
Children*, 47, 3,
228–9.

Improving attitudes of high school students towards their handicapped peers

Description of an experimental eight-week educational programme to enable high school students to become more knowledgeable about handicapped people and to ease the mainstreaming of handicapped children into class. The young people discussed terminology and laws; researched and reported on specific disabilities; watched a film about the handicapped; tried out simulation activities to experience what handicaps felt like; and talked to a blind student. Afterwards, 82 per cent said they felt that their attitudes had become more positive and accepting. A majority rated direct contact with the handicapped person as the most effective part of the scheme. The experiment was considered a success and was adopted for young people taking the sociology course.

O'MOORE, M.
(1980)
*Child: Care,
Health and
Development*, 6,
6, 317–37.

Social acceptance of the physically handicapped child in the ordinary school

Thirty-eight visibly handicapped children aged 9 to 11 who attended ordinary schools in Scotland were studied to see whether they were accepted by their schoolmates. Over half the children were cerebral palsied. The handicapped children were matched with able-bodied control children; all children were of normal intelligence. Social acceptance of the physically handicapped by schoolmates was assessed by a social discrimination questionnaire asking about who should play popular and unpopular parts in an imaginary film. Two tests also assessed the children's emotional adjustment, and the visibility of the handicap was rated on a 4-point scale.

The average social acceptance score for the handicapped group was −4.55, and the average score for the controls was +4.70 – a highly significant difference. When the two groups of children were ranked for popularity, the handicapped children were ranked significantly below the control children. Acceptance or rejection was not related to the severity of the disability or to its visual impression, but it was related to intelligence and school ability. Popularity was clearly correlated with extraversion and with good emotional and social adjustment, for both groups of children. Teachers underestimated the unpopularity of the handicapped, although they did estimate that they were teased more frequently than the control children. It is recommended that children in ordinary schools be educated to understand and accept disability.

ALTMAN, B.M.
(1981)
Social Problems,
28, 3, 321–37.

Studies of attitudes towards the handicapped: the need for a new direction

A review article of studies published over the past 25 years, with nearly 100 references. It is suggested that more research should be done on adult attitudes rather than children's, and especially those of people in positions of influence, such as employers, bank managers and police. The effect of educational 'mainstreaming' of handicapped children should be investigated. Attitudes are complex and multi-dimensional and future research should take account of this.

ROSENBAUM,
P.L. and
ARMSTRONG,
R.W.
(1984)
Paper presented
at annual
convention of the
American
Psychological
Association in
Toronto, Canada.

Changing children's attitudes towards disabled peers: randomized controlled trials of buddy and educational programs

An account of three studies in changing children's attitudes carried out in Canada. In the first, children in grades 5 to 8 were asked if they would be a 'buddy' to a handicapped child; over half agreed. Their attitudes to handicap were first tested on a specially constructed questionnaire; then 42 children were randomly chosen and paired with a handicapped child for weekly non-academic activities for three months. The handicapped children were quite severely disabled, mainly by cerebral palsy or spina bifida. At the end of the three months, the 42 children, together with a control group who had not been 'buddies', were tested again on their attitudes. The 'buddies' had significantly more positive attitudes than the control group.

The second study used a puppet show relating to various handicaps. This was shown to schoolchildren once a week for ten weeks. Some children acted as 'buddies', some were 'buddies' and also saw the puppet programmes, and some were involved in neither activity. Although the attitude scores of the 'buddies' improved, those of the children who both acted as 'buddies' and also saw the puppet shows did not; it is suggested that the two programmes were not compatible with one another. The third study used only the puppet shows, and found that they had no effect on attitudes. The authors recommend extension of the 'buddy' type of experiment, but point out that only the children who had consented to it were involved. It would be valuable to know what the impact would be on children who refuse.

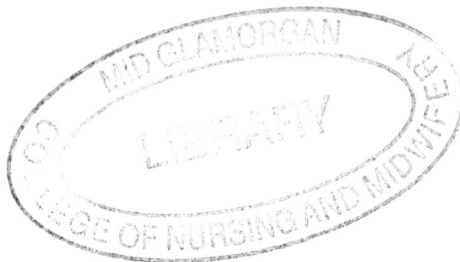

SECTION II

Emotional and Social Adjustment

There can be little doubt that emotional disorder is more common among cerebral palsied children than among the non-handicapped. While this has long been suggested by those who work with cerebral palsied children, actual research evidence is fairly recent. There are two studies that have compared prevalence rates of psychiatric disorder in cerebral palsied children with those for non-handicapped children. Nielsen (1966) compared 40 spastic children (IQs above 75) with normal children, matched for age, sex and intelligence, and found that significantly more of the spastic children showed signs of moderate or severe disorder on one of three projective tests. The validity of these tests has, however, been questioned by Rutter, Graham and Yule (1970a). Their own study, though, using a psychiatric interview for selected children and teachers' and parental questionnaires, found a very much higher rate of psychiatric disorder (47.9 per cent) among schoolchildren with brain lesions (mostly with cerebral palsy) on the Isle of Wight than among either non-handicapped children (6.6 per cent) or physically handicapped children without brain involvement (11.6 per cent). A third study (McMichael, 1971a) assessed maladjustment by comparing the rate of child guidance clinic referral in a school for the physically handicapped with the rate for ordinary schools, finding it to be nearly three times as high.

In two recent studies Anderson (1973) (see Section IV) and Anderson et al. (1982) have investigated the position of handicapped children in both ordinary schools and special schools and, among other factors, assessed social and emotional adjustment. In the earlier study, physically handicapped children's adjustment to ordinary schools is examined. Those children among the handicapped who had neurological abnormalities, such as cerebral palsy, were found to have a higher rate of behaviour disorder than the other handicapped children. In the 1982 study Anderson and her associates were concerned with adolescents with cerebral palsy and spina bifida. Psychological problems were considered to be present in about half the handicapped children – a much higher rate than among the non-handicapped. In Anderson's two studies there is also a wealth of information about the school problems – popularity, social life – of the cerebral palsied.

A higher proportion, then, of cerebral palsied children than normal children do have psychiatric disorders; but there is little evidence to support the suggestion that they have a specific type of psychiatric disorder. In the Isle of Wight study (Rutter, Graham and

9

Yule, 1970a) it was found that the majority of children with brain lesions (excluding those under the mental subnormality services) had neurotic or antisocial disorders, as do children in the general population who have psychiatric disorders. This study also compared the prevalence of individual items of behaviour often attributed to brain damage – such as high or low motor activity, fidgetiness, poor concentration, irritability – in the neuro-epileptic and general population. While a high rate of such characteristics was found in the neuro-epileptic population, the majority were also found frequently among the non-neurologically handicapped children with psychiatric disorders. For two items, reduced motor activity and poor concentration, there did appear to be an association (though not a very strong one) with organic brain defect. For most of the characteristics, though, that are attributed to brain damage the association seems to be with psychiatric disorder rather than with the neurological defect itself. Miller (1958) from a study of children attending a child guidance clinic in New York found that the difficulties of mildly handicapped cerebral palsied children, within the normal range of intelligence, were exactly the same as those of physically and neurologically normal children, except for additional problems in perception and concept formation.

The position appears to be rather different in the severely mentally subnormal (IQ below 50) for these children, whether or not they had cerebral palsy, showed a high rate of psychiatric disorder in the Isle of Wight study (Graham, Rutter and Yule, 1970a) and the hyperkinetic syndrome and psychosis were much more frequent than in the general population.

The question arises as to how much of the behaviour disorder found in cerebral palsied children is due to the neurological abnormality itself and how much to the strain of having to grow up with a visible and frustrating handicap. Oswin (1967) has described the kind of problems cerebral palsied children have to struggle with, and several papers (Miller, 1958; Minde *et al.*, 1972; Minde, 1978; Teplin *et al.*, 1981) have discussed the developing self-concept of cerebral palsied children as they grow up to try to make a place for themselves in the world. Minde and his colleagues found the children understandably very prone to bouts of depression. Muthard (1965) and Freeman (1970) both give it as their opinion that problems are attributed to brain damage which are in fact a result of life experience.

This difficult life experience does make a contribution to the high rate of psychiatric disorder in cerebral palsied children, therefore. Nevertheless the work by Rutter, Graham and Yule (1970a) makes it clear that an overriding factor is the brain dysfunction itself. From comparison with a group of children having lesions below the brain stem (mainly with post-poliomyelitis or muscular dystrophy), who had severe and obvious physical defects but a much lower rate of psychiatric disorder, it appeared that neither the severity nor the visibility of the physical handicap or social prejudice could account for the increased rate of psychiatric disorder in the cerebral palsied. Low intelligence was an important factor but even when intelligence was controlled the neuro-epileptic children still had more psychiatric disorder than the other physically handicapped children. The authors conclude that the brain dysfunction itself is the most important feature in the high rate of psychiatric disorder. This is confirmed by the work of Seidel *et al.* (1975), who compared a group of children with neurological disorders with a group with handicaps such as muscular dystrophy. The brain-injured children were found to have twice as high a rate of psychiatric disorder as the crippled children without brain injury.

Seidel and his colleagues found psychiatric disorder to be associated with broken or unhappy homes and with a mother who had psychiatric problems. Because of this, and because a majority of the neurologically damaged were *not* psychiatrically disturbed, and because there was no specific form of psychiatric syndrome, they point out that brain damage does not lead directly to psychiatric illness but merely increases the child's vulnerability to it. Rutter, Graham and Yule also suggest that while the child with a brain disorder is more susceptible to psychiatric disturbance than other children, many of the factors which actually cause the disorder to occur are the same as in any other children.

Finally, a number of studies touch on the cerebral palsied child's social relationships, particularly at school (Ingram *et al.*, 1964a; Nielsen, 1966; Anderson, 1973 (see Section IV); O'Moore, 1980 (see Section I); Margalit, 1981; Anderson *et al.*, 1982; Madge and Fassam, 1982). All show that the cerebral palsied child has a restricted life compared to his or her non-handicapped peers, which is perhaps inevitable; several of these authors feel that the cerebral palsied could be encouraged to be less passive, however. The studies found a tendency for the cerebral palsied to be less popular than average at school, and to have friends mainly among other handicapped children. It was also noted (Anderson *et al.*, 1982) that disabled teenagers knew very little about their handicap, and communicated little with their parents about it.

It seems then that many children with cerebral palsy, in addition to physical, intellectual and sensory problems, are also burdened with emotional and social difficulties.

MILLER, E.A.
(1958)
*Exceptional
Children*, 24, 7,
298–302; 305.

Cerebral palsied children and their parents

Findings are reported from clinical experience with 55 children, of dull normal to high average intelligence, who attended a child guidance clinic in New York. The 26 mildly handicapped cerebral palsied children, referred to the clinic with severe behaviour and learning problems, were educationally retarded by one to three years below mental age (on standardized tests), their self-concept showed feelings of physical and mental inadequacy and self-abasement (on projective tests), they showed anxiety and insecurity in relationships with parents, many had an unusual amount of hostility and most (80 per cent) had problems of perception and concept formation.

The difficulties of 13 physically and neurologically normal children, matched in age, intelligence and referral reasons with the cerebral palsied group, were indistinguishable from those of the physically handicapped children except that they did not have problems of perception and concept formation. The 16 severely handicapped cerebral palsied children could not be evaluated on all measures but the predominant finding from projective tests (eight tested) was of excessive dependence and immaturity.

Parents of the mildly cerebral palsied children were confused about the child's capabilities – they reacted with anxiety, over-expectation and had negative feelings resulting from frustration. Parents of the physically normal children had very similar feelings, but showed more overt hostility. In contrast, parents of the severely handicapped children were much more accepting but encouraged dependence. Individual therapy with the available mildly handicapped (14 lived too far away) and physically normal children, and with their parents, showed a high rate of success (22 out of 25) and gains held on re-evaluation one to four years later. Only three of the mildly handicapped untreated children showed positive changes on re-evaluation.

SMALL, J.G.
(1962)
*Archives of
General
Psychiatry*, 7, 2,
120–4.

A psychiatric survey of brain-injured children

131 children (66 with cerebral palsy) who attended a clinic for children with cerebral palsy and language disorders, attached to the University of Oregon Medical School, were evaluated psychiatrically and their parents interviewed. One-third (45) of the children were found to have specific psychiatric difficulties, but 25 of these did not display the type of behaviour problems (hyperkinetic behaviour syndrome) usually considered to denote an organic basis. Among the cerebral palsied children, one-sixth (11) were found to have psychiatric disorders (five cases possibly

having an organic origin). In the group as a whole, psychiatric disorders tended to be related to severe hearing or visual defects, older age (only 10 per cent of the under six age group but nearly 60 per cent of the over 12 age group showed emotional disturbances) and to psychiatric difficulties in the parents.

INGRAM, T.T.S., JAMESON, S., ERRINGTON, J. and MITCHELL, R.G. (1964a) Clinics in Developmental Medicine no.14. London: Spastics Society in association with Heinemann. (Especially Chapter 4, 'Social life and personal relationships'.)

Living with Cerebral Palsy

A follow-up study of 200 adolescents and young adults, born between 1938 and 1947, and originally included in surveys of the cerebral palsied in the eastern region of Scotland (Henderson, 1961 – see Cockburn, 1961a (see Section III)). Subjects were grouped into seven categories according to the type of social life they had. Groups ranged from those leading a relatively normal social life (21 per cent), a restricted social life (25 per cent) to those who never left the house for social activities (4 per cent) and those in institutions for the mentally handicapped (12 per cent).

70 per cent of those with a mild handicap were in the first two categories, being accepted by their contemporaries on equal terms, against 25 per cent of those with moderate or severe handicaps. 81 per cent of those with average intelligence were in these two categories. Severity of physical handicap, more than level of intelligence, was important in finding friends outside the family.

Although 186 of the subjects were of marriageable age, only four were married, compared with the 19.4 per cent for males and 33.4 per cent for females that would have been expected if the subjects had not been handicapped. Subjects were very aware of their disadvantages in attracting the opposite sex – they not only tended to look less attractive but also had less well-paid jobs, if they were employed – compared with the non-handicapped of their own age.

MUTHARD, J.E. (1965) *Journal of Consulting Psychology*, 29, 6, 599.

MMPI findings for cerebral palsied college students

As part of an investigation of cerebral palsied college students (see Muthard and Hutchison, 1968 (Section IV)), the Minnesota Multiphasic Personality Inventory (MMPI) was used to measure personality differences between the cerebral palsied and non-handicapped students. The students with cerebral palsy showed greater emotional disturbance and were more in need of psychological help. Differences appeared to be due, in part, to the actual difficulties arising from the handicap rather than from personality deviations. The men cerebral palsied students showed greater degrees of worry, feelings of worthlessness and seclusiveness than the women. There were no significant personality differences between the mildly, moderately and severely handicapped.

NIELSEN, H.H.
(1966)
Copenhagen:
Munksgaard.
(Especially Part I,
Chapters 3 and 5;
Part II, Chapters
6, 9 and 10.)

A Psychological Study of Cerebral Palsied Children

Part I reviews the research literature on cerebral palsied children, including that on intelligence, cognitive and visual-motor functions and personality. Part II reports a psychological study of 40 spastic children with IQs of 75 or more who were attending an out-patient clinic of the University Hospital of Copenhagen. Twenty-one were mildly handicapped, nine moderately and ten moderately severely. Comparisons were made with a control group of 40 normal children.

In the analysis of personality, significantly more of the spastic children than the controls showed signs of moderate or severe disorder on one of three projective tests (Thematic Apperception Test, Duss Fable Test, Rorschach). Nevertheless only seven spastic children (as against two controls) showed signs of personality disorder on all three tests. More disorders were found among the hemiplegic than among the paraplegic children. Age, sex, and degree of handicap did not affect the results but those with IQs below 90 were most likely to be emotionally disturbed.

The most common problems in the spastic children were that they experienced difficulties in personal relationships, expected hostility and rejection, were more easily emotionally aroused than normal children and responded to frustration with aggression and defiance. Information about the spastic children's home and school adjustment was obtained from parents and teachers. In general the adolescent worried more about his or her handicap than the younger child. While the parents' attitude was of great importance, there did not appear to be as close a relationship between home environment and the child's emotional adjustment as in normal children. About a third of the children had difficulties in relationships with normal children; some were timid and anxious, others aggressive and domineering. Half of the children at ordinary schools were rated as average in academic attainments and concentration, despite almost three-quarters being slow workers.

OSWIN, M.
(1967)
Bristol: John
Wright and Sons.

Behaviour Problems Amongst Children with Cerebral Palsy

Description of the kinds of emotional problems found in children with cerebral palsy – and of how these may arise from the effects of physical, sensory or perceptual handicaps, from 'broken' homes, rejecting or over-protective parents or from the insecurity and lack of normal experiences in institutional care. Ways in which the teacher may alleviate the child's problems are discussed. Case histories are used extensively as illustrations.

FREEMAN, R.D.
(1970)
*Developmental
Medicine and
Child Neurology*,
12, 64–70.

Psychiatric problems in adolescents with cerebral palsy

There is a lack of research data on emotional problems in cerebral palsy and the author bases the discussion on his six years of clinical experience in the field, as well as on the experience of others. Problems often attributed to brain damage may, in fact, be due to the life experience of the handicapped. At adolescence handicaps take on a different meaning for the patient and his or her family. Handicaps may hinder fulfilment of the adolescent's social, sexual and vocational needs. Indirect psychiatric help through the parents may be the most effective way of solving problems, although individual psychotherapy, group or family therapy, behaviour modification techniques and drug therapy may all be of use in particular cases.

RUTTER, M.,
GRAHAM, P. and
YULE, W.
(1970a)
Clinics in
Developmental
Medicine no.
35/36. London:
Spastics
International
Medical
Publications in
association with
Heinemann.
(Especially Part
IV.)

A Neuropsychiatric Study in Childhood

In this study of all school-age children with neuro-epileptic disorders living on the Isle of Wight, the rate of psychiatric disorder was much higher among the children with brain lesions, most of whom had cerebral palsy (58.3 per cent in those with fits and 37.5 per cent in those without fits) than it was in 10- to 11-year-old normal (6.6 per cent) or physically handicapped (11.6 per cent) children. The main factor associated with this higher rate of psychiatric disorder appeared to be the presence of a dysfunction in the brain itself. The difference in the rates of the children with brain lesions and the other physically handicapped children could not be accounted for by differences in severity of the physical handicap, its visibility or social rejection.

Although there was an association between low intelligence and psychiatric disorder, even in the group of neuro-epileptic children with IQs of 86+ the rate of psychiatric disorder was twice as high as it was amongst the physically handicapped children without brain involvement. The types of psychiatric disorder, though, were similar among both children with and without brain disorder, consisting mainly of neurotic and antisocial disorders. Certain items of behaviour, such as restlessness, poor concentration and irritability, have been associated by many researchers with brain damage. Although these types of behaviour were more common in the neuro-epileptic group than in the general population, they were mostly found as often in the children with psychiatric disorders but no brain lesions as in the children with both psychiatric and brain disorders. The exceptions were a tendency for there to be an association between neuro-epileptic disorder and reduced motor activity, and for an even slighter association with poor concentration.

In contrast to the lack of association between specific types of psychiatric disorder and brain damage in children with IQs above 50, amongst severely subnormal children (including those with cerebral palsy and other definite brain lesions), over half of those with psychiatric disorder showed either the hyperkinetic syndrome or psychosis. Within the group of children with structural brain disorders and IQs of 50+, psychiatric disorders appeared to be associated with bilateral rather than unilateral brain disorder, strabismus, language retardation; low IQ and specific reading retardation, 'broken' homes and emotional disturbance in the mother.

It seems that while neuro-epileptic children are more vulnerable to psychiatric disorder than other children, the factors associated with psychiatric disorder are the same as in non-handicapped children. While the children with brain disorders appeared to be less socially acceptable to other children than asthmatic children, this was related to the high rate of psychiatric disorder in the group rather than to the type of handicap.

McMICHAEL, J.K. (1971a) London: Staples Press. (Especially Chapters 6 and 8.)

Handicap: A Study of Physically Handicapped Children and Their Families

In 50 children attending a school for the physically handicapped in the London area (21 children had cerebral palsy, eight post-polio disabilities and 21 various other handicaps) the rate of referral for clinic guidance was 24 per cent, three times the rate for ordinary schools (as reported by the Underwood Committee). From parental and teacher assessments 44 per cent of the children were judged to show normal or slight emotional difficulties in adjustment to their handicap and 56 per cent moderate to severe difficulties. The main factor determining the children's emotional adjustment was parental attitudes.

MINDE, K.K.,
HACKETT, J.D.,
KILLOU, D., and
SILVER, S.
(1972)
*American Journal
of Psychiatry*, 128,
1554–60.

How they grow up: 41 physically handicapped children and their families

A follow-up study of 41 children from a special day school in Montreal aged five to nine years. About half had IQ scores below 80. Parents were given long interviews, children and school staff were also interviewed, and teachers rated the children's emotional adjustment twice a year on the Rutter scale.

Regarding the children's schooling, it was found that many of them had reacted with distress to being away from home in the day, but had recovered within the first six months. Parents had at first been pleased and hopeful about the school placement, but after a time both parent and child had begun to realize the limits of what the school could do. In addition, as the children grew older they lost their non-handicapped playmates and only had friends among their handicapped schoolmates. Twelve of the 41 children, most of them of average intelligence, consequently had had crises of depression lasting from weeks to a year. Among the non-retarded group, a few were starting to envisage the future with their handicap, while most of the retarded children appeared not to think about it.

Where the child's future was concerned, parents fell into two categories: one, larger, group felt that the child must get used to being 'different' and envisaged a very limited future, while the other group determined the child must be part of the community and had optimistic future plans. There was no significant difference, in the children of these two groups of parents, in intelligence or extent of handicap, but the non-handicapped siblings in the high-expectancy group had more problems, especially of jealousy, than those from the other group. The authors conclude that between five and nine the handicapped child may begin to realize that his or her handicap is permanent, to go through a depression, and then to begin to adjust. The parents appear to be torn between acknowledging the normal and the abnormal aspects of their children and to tend to emphasize one or the other. Professionals must work towards establishing a secure place for the handicapped person in the community.

BATTLE, C.U.
(1974)
*Rehabilitation
Literature*, 35, 5,
130–40.

Disruptions in the socialization of a young, severely handicapped child

A review of the various and complex ways in which any handicapped child – particularly the one with cerebral palsy – may be affected by his or her disability throughout growing up and socialization. Early care may be in the hands of a depressed mother, and may be interrupted by hospitalizations. If the handicapped baby is unresponsive it may be difficult for the mother to act warmly. In early childhood, the child's interaction with the environment is distorted; independence may be particularly hard to foster. The lack of a peer group and the absence of play are major deprivations, and once at school he or she may feel different and inferior. Everything possible must be done to help parents overcome these problems, in particular by providing sensory experience.

PODEANU-
CZEHOFSKY, I.
(1975)
*Rehabilitation
Literature*, 36, 10,
308–11.

Is it only the child's guilt? Some aspects of family life of cerebral palsied children

From an Austrian hospital concerned with the rehabilitation of cerebral palsied children, 65 patients were studied. The author comes to the conclusion that within the family the handicapped child's adjustment is no different from that of his or her siblings and that it is outside the home that difficulties arise. Problems of some kind were found in 80 per cent of her sample – parental conflict, broken homes, rejection or over-indulgence of the child. More attention should be paid to the psychological difficulties of handicapped children, rather than to physical difficulties alone.

SEIDEL, U.P.,
CHADWICK,
O.F.D., and
RUTTER, M.
(1975)
*Developmental
Medicine and
Child Neurology*,
17, 5, 563–73.

Psychological disorders in crippled children. A comparative study of children with and without brain damage

In order to assess the role of brain damage in psychiatric disturbance, crippled children aged between 5 and 14 from three London boroughs were assessed. All children had an IQ of 70 or above. The sample was divided into two groups: 33 children with a disorder due to brain injury, and 42 with a disorder due to some other cause (polio, muscular dystrophy, etc.). The groups were similar in age, sex, social class, and severity of handicap. Psychiatric disorder was assessed by interviewing parents, teachers and children.

The brain-injured children were found to have twice as high a rate of psychiatric disorder as the crippled children without brain injury. Brain damage was also associated with reading backwardness and low intelligence. Social class and family size were not related to psychiatric disorder, but it was significantly more common in children from overcrowded homes, broken homes, from families with marital discord, or where there was a mother who had psychiatric problems. It is concluded that brain damage was responsible for the children's increased vulnerability to emotional problems. Nevertheless, it is pointed out that three-quarters of the brain-damaged children did not have emotional problems, and also that there was no specific type of emotional disorder associated with brain damage; therefore it seems clear that the brain damage did not lead *directly* to psychiatric problems, but merely increased the child's vulnerability to psycho-social hazards.

CRUICKSHANK,
W.M. and BICE,
H.V.
(1976)
In:
CRUICKSHANK,
W.M. (Ed)
*Cerebral Palsy: a
Developmental
Disability.*
Revised edition.
Syracuse:
Syracuse
University Press,
pp. 135–91.

Personality characteristics

The emotional adjustment of the cerebral palsied child and adolescent is discussed in relation to: (1) the social situation – parental and community attitudes; (2) self-concept of the cerebral palsied; and (3) perceptual difficulties. The authors draw on their own and others' research findings and their clinical experience.

MINDE, K.K.
(1978)
*American Journal
of Psychiatry*, 135,
1344–9.

Coping style of 34 adolescents with cerebral palsy

A follow-up study of cerebral palsied adolescents in Montreal first studied in childhood (see p.17). The sample comprised 34 young people between 12 and 15, of whom 23 were still attending a special school and 11 were at ordinary schools. All were moderately or severely physically handicapped but in the educable intelligence range. Parents, teachers and the young people themselves were all interviewed for the follow-up, and psychiatric assessments were made using the ratings devised by Rutter. The adolescents were also asked about their feelings and aspirations.
Parents tended to be less hopeful about their children's futures than they had been earlier, and less likely to seek discussion or advice. Of the 19 families who had other children beside the cerebral palsied one, 14 said that the non-handicapped siblings had suffered because of the situation. In general parents had little idea of what the children felt about their handicap. The parents' concern was now more about schooling problems than about emotional adjustment. The young people themselves

talked openly about their handicap and understood some of its consequences. Their plans for the future were uncertain, but more of the children at ordinary schools than at special schools had definite ideas about future careers. About a third of them all now had some non-handicapped friends. 18 per cent were assessed as having definite psychiatric disturbance; this was closely correlated with parental discord, and also with having no non-handicapped friends.

The author feels that the main themes in the children's development were greater understanding of the permanence of the handicap, and a precarious search for an occupational identity. There were indications that the first signs of passivity and low self-esteem were appearing.

MARGALIT, M. (1981) *Israel Journal of Psychiatry and Rehabilitation Sciences*, 18, 3, 209–14.

Leisure activities of cerebral palsy children

The leisure activities of 51 cerebral palsied children in Israel were compared with those of a group of 20 able-bodied children. The age range of the children was 9 to 17, and for all of them intelligence was in the normal range. The cerebral palsied children were all at a special school and their degree of physical handicap varied – some were in wheelchairs. All the children were asked about their leisure activities, including titles of books read and films seen, and types of excursions.

The cerebral palsied children read significantly fewer books than the control children, and the choice of them reflected adult guidance. Viewing of television and listening to radio was similar for the two groups. Youth club activity was more restricted for the cerebral palsied group. Spontaneous social activities were rare among the cerebral palsied group. The cerebral palsied rarely went to films, and when they did go it was with parents, to films of the parents' choice; the same applied to excursions. In general, the handicapped group's activities were mostly taken with the family and were planned and chosen by others rather than by themselves, encouraging a passive life style and delaying maturity. It is suggested that a major effort be made to integrate handicapped children into young people's activities.

TEPLIN, S.W.,
HOWARD, J.A.,
and O'CONNOR,
M.J.
(1981)
*Developmental
Medicine and
Child Neurology,*
23, 6, 730–8.

Self-concept of young children with cerebral palsy

The self-concepts of 15 cerebral palsied children aged four to eight, of normal intelligence and middle-class background and attending ordinary schools in California, were compared with those of 15 matched children without handicap. The children all completed a specially designed test, and parents and teachers filled in a rating scale for self-concept. There was only a non-significant tendency for the cerebral palsied children to have a lower self-concept, but teachers – not parents – rated the cerebral palsied children as having lower self-esteem than the other group. The authors suggest that cerebral palsied children begin to regard themselves as 'different' as early as four years old, but the negative effect on self-esteem does not begin until later.

ANDERSON,
E.M., CLARKE,
L., and SPAIN, B.
(1982)
London:
Methuen.

Disability in Adolescence

119 handicapped adolescents aged 15 to 19 were surveyed, 89 of them with cerebral palsy and 30 with spina bifida and hydrocephalus. Most had further handicaps such as epilepsy, speech defect or incontinence. All had IQs of 70 or over. 31 per cent were at ordinary schools and the rest at special schools. For part of the study, a control group of non-handicapped teenagers from the same school was studied for comparison. The teenagers, their parents, and school staff were all interviewed, and 51 of the teenagers were followed up for a year after leaving school.

Independence and responsibility: It was felt that parents could have allowed the young people more independence. It was noticeable that the majority knew little about their handicaps and had never spoken to a medically trained person about it. Information on benefits and allowances was also scanty.

Leisure activities: The handicapped teenagers went out less and viewed more television, but they also read fewer books and newspapers.

Friendships: The handicapped teenagers, more often than controls, were described by teachers as being 'somewhat disliked', and by parents as being shy and withdrawn. There was no evidence that they were teased much more than other children, however. There was as much teasing at special schools as at the ordinary schools. Far fewer of the handicapped teenagers met friends outside school hours; frequency of meetings was related to mobility and to severity of handicap. Fewer of the handicapped than controls had special friends, and fewer went out in a group. All the young people were rated ('satisfactory', 'limited' or 'very restricted') on their social life, and over 90 per cent of the controls had a satisfactory social life as compared to 21 per cent of the handicapped. Restriction increased with the severity of the handicap.

Relations with the opposite sex: The handicapped teenagers had little opportunity to go out with the opposite sex, and they worried about this more than their parents realized. Nearly all wanted to marry and have children, but were uncertain whether they would be able to.

Psychological adjustment: problems were considered to be present in about half the handicapped teenagers, i.e. much more commonly than in the control group, and they were generally of the neurotic rather than the antisocial type – depression, anxiety and lack of confidence. Epilepsy, incontinence and low intelligence were all associated with psychological problems, as was the presence of mental health problems in the mother.

Post-school placements of the handicapped after one year: 56 per cent of those leaving special schools had no qualifications, and 17 per cent of those leaving ordinary schools. After school 33 per cent were in employment, 26 per cent in further education, 20 per cent in a day centre and 22 per cent at home; the most contented were those in further education, and those at home or in day centres were very dissatisfied.

Stress after leaving school: The handicapped teenagers were distressed by delays in placement, lack of activity, and justifiable anxiety about the future. 40 per cent suffered from severe social isolation, and some had problems within the family as well. Only half could use a bus unaccompanied, and a quarter had driving licences. Depression was common. Few schools had offered counselling or vocational guidance. The teenagers were mostly not able to discuss their handicap with parents or peers.

Conclusions: The authors emphasize four main points: the inadequacy of the handicapped young people's social life; the lack of control they experienced over their lives, and the lack of discussion and information; the poverty of choice for those unable to find work, and the limitations of day centres; the lack of preparation and vocational guidance for adult life.

MADGE, N. and
FASSAM, M.
(1982)
London: Batsford
Academic

Ask the Children

Four groups of children were studied: 46 from a school for the disabled (aged 6–15), and 13 disabled pupils at ordinary schools (aged 11–17); as control groups, 13 able-bodied matched children from a comprehensive school and 16 able-bodied children from a primary school. One-third of the disabled children were cerebral palsied, and other handicaps included spina bifida, muscular dystrophy, etc. The children were given open-ended interviews on disability, education, social life, family life and future plans, and their answers are quoted in detail.

Attitudes towards disability: Few except the oldest of the handicapped children knew much about their condition and its causes, and few reported much opportunity to talk about it or ask questions. When they were asked about the problems of their disability, the majority mentioned physical limitations, but 18 per cent mentioned problems in mixing and making friends.

Education: Among both disabled and well children, more positive than negative comments were made about school, and all groups mentioned the same kind of likes and dislikes. Just over a quarter said they would like to go to a different school. On the whole the children who had transferred from the special school to the comprehensive were glad they had moved, although many had had difficulties at first. When the children were asked about the merits of integrated versus special schooling, it was the pupils who had transferred to the comprehensive who were most in favour of integrated schooling.

Friends and social life: Most of the able-bodied children had friends at their own and other schools, while the disabled had friends only in their own school. Over half the disabled had friends among the able-bodied, but there was a minority who suffered from difficulty in making friends due to lack of social skills. Nearly two-thirds of the able-bodied seniors thought handicapped children were likely to be teased, and over half the handicapped reported teasing. The able-bodied had more leisure activities than the disabled.

Family and home life: There was no evidence that the families with a handicapped child were more split by divorce than the control families. More of the disabled than the able-bodied were only children or firstborn. Disabled children were less likely than controls to go out with friends and more likely to go on outings with parents. There was no evidence that they got on worse with siblings than the control children did. Some of the disabled children spent a lot of time at home watching television or playing records.

Plans for the future: Disabled children were more likely than control children to look forward to leaving school, but they had less definite ideas about the future than the others. Among the disabled children both at the special school and the comprehensive there were at least a third who were unrealistic or blank about future plans. Only half the disabled senior children said they hoped to marry and have children.

SECTION III
Family Adjustment

The importance of parental attitudes and psychological stability in the emotional adjustment of physically handicapped children is well recognized. Rutter, Graham and Yule, 1970a (see Section II) stress that while neurological features may make the cerebral palsied child particularly susceptible to emotional disorder, the influence of emotional factors in the home is still very important. While opinions range on the effect of parental attitudes on the cerebral palsied child from those of McMichael, 1971a (see Section II) who suggests they are the key factor (for all physically handicapped children) to those of Nielsen, 1966 (see Section II) who thinks they have somewhat less influence than in the normal child, there can be no doubt that they do play an essential role in the child's emotional development.

Studies of parental attitudes in the cerebral palsied child's family fall into two groups: there are those that look for parental pathology and tend to see most parents of the handicapped as candidates for psychiatric counselling (Boles, 1959; Jensen and Kogan, 1962; Adams, 1968; McMichael, 1971b); and those that start from the premise that these parents are no different from other couples except that they are called on to carry an exceptional burden of difficulties (Carnegie United Kingdom Trust, 1964; Bowley, 1967 (see Section IV); Hewett, 1970; Glendinning, 1983).

Among the former, McMichael, in her study of parents of children with various physical handicaps, found a high rate of rejection (31 per cent), over-protection (46 per cent) and overall failure to adjust (56 per cent). Boles (1959) also found a high rate of anxiety, guilt, rejection, unrealistic attitudes and social withdrawal; but in his control group of mothers of non-handicapped children there were similar rates, according to his criteria. It is doubtful, therefore, whether parents of the handicapped differ from average in these respects. A point on which several studies do agree (Boles, 1959; Jensen and Kogan, 1962; Barclay and Vaught, 1964; Keith and Markie, 1969; Minde et al., 1971) is that, while parents are realistic about the present, they find it difficult to be equally realistic about their child's future; but, as Keith and Markie suggest, optimism is necessary to sustain parents who have to remain responsible for a handicapped child over many years.

Two studies approach the question of family difficulties more sensitively. Kogan et al. (1974) examined the interaction of a small sample of mothers with their cerebral palsied children, and found that during the child's early years warm and positive behaviour decreased in the mother; the same, however, was true of the children's physiotherapists. It may be that what is classified as rejection is rather a closing down of inappropriate hopes, especially for a child that will never walk. In a very different type of study Schaffer (1964) has isolated a type of family functioning that he found in 13 out of 30 families with a cerebral palsied child: the 'too-cohesive' family, which centres round the handicapped member and closes up against the outside world.

If this is one way of coping with the care of a handicapped child, it might be expected sometimes to have an adverse effect on siblings. Morgenstern (1966) found siblings of 30 cerebral palsied children to be more emotionally unstable than children in a control group; on the other hand, several studies (Carnegie United Kingdom Trust, 1964; Hewett, 1970; Lloyd-Bostock, 1976) concluded that siblings of the cerebral palsied child were not affected for the worse by the existence of their handicapped brother or sister. Breslau *et al.* (1981) found that, overall, siblings were no more disturbed than control children, though they had higher scores on some items of the inventory used. The evidence, as discussed in a review article by Simeonsson and McHale (1981) is contradictory; no doubt there are both gains and losses for siblings of any handicapped child.

Turning to the studies which find the more positive qualities in the families of the cerebral palsied, Bowley (1967) (listed under Section IV) found that the great majority of parents of educable children who had received early education and treatment at the Cheyne Centre for Spastic Children were 'realistic, affectionate and constructive' towards their children. Lloyd-Bostock (1976) cites similar qualities of love and appreciation for their handicapped child in a sample of parents (these were mentally handicapped children, but not necessarily cerebral palsied). Hewett (1970) argues that in any case judgements about parents' 'acceptance' of the child's handicap are irrelevant. In her very thorough study of 180 mothers of cerebral palsied children she found that child-rearing methods were much the same as in families with normal children, except for the obvious allowances having to be made for handicap.

Hewett, as well as Lloyd-Bostock, Minde *et al.* (1971) and Glendinning (1983), presents a picture of parents coping with anxiety and strain which is increased by the inadequacy of services provided for them. Many parents in Lloyd-Bostock's sample had had a long struggle to get their children diagnosed and suitably placed. The title of Glendinning's book, *Unshared Care*, speaks for itself; the families she investigated had had similar problems, and were not made aware of the services that could be made available. About half of the parents in Tarran's (1981) sample in Scotland were dissatisfied with the information they had been given and wanted more discussion. These studies, mostly relying on long interviews rather than pencil-and-paper tests, give the impression of parents coping valiantly with problems, with all too little help.

BOLES, G.
(1959)
Genetic
Psychology
Monographs, 59,
2, 159–218.

Personality factors in mothers of cerebral palsied children

Mothers of cerebral palsied children were found to be more overprotective and to have more conflicts in their marriage relationships than mothers of non-handicapped children. The two groups did not differ in anxiety, guilt, rejection, unrealistic attitudes or social withdrawal, but these characteristics were found in a high proportion of mothers in both groups. Mothers of the children with cerebral palsy were realistic about their child's present functioning and lack of social opportunities, but unrealistic about his or her future achievements. Subjects (60 mothers of cerebral palsied children and 60 mothers of non-handicapped children, from the New York area, the two groups being matched on ten variables including religion, socio-economic status, age of mother and age of child) were administered a questionnaire with ten sub-scales to examine their attitudes, feelings and behaviour.

COCKBURN, J.
(1961a)
In: HENDERSON,
J.L. (Ed) *Cerebral
Palsy in
Childhood and
Adolescence. A
Medical,
Psychological and
Social Study.*
Edinburgh and
London: E. and S.
Livingstone, pp.
281–324. (Section
on 'Psychological
aspects of the
home'.)

Psychological and educational aspects

As part of a survey of the cerebral palsied children and adolescents, up to the age of 21, living in the eastern region of Scotland, the subjects' homes were visited. Of the 223 homes, about a quarter were considered unsuitable for a handicapped person, either because of psychological or material difficulties which were usually unconnected with the cerebral palsied child himself. The handicap was usually better understood in homes of good intellectual level, and where the child was older and the handicap more severe, but acceptance was not related to these factors. The IQ of the cerebral palsied child was related to the intellectual status of the home. About a fifth of the homes failed to provide stimulation for the child. Parents differed greatly in the type of problems, resulting from the handicap, which concerned them most. Problems were mainly those which would have arisen at the child's age anyway, but were possibly exacerbated by the handicap. Where the handicap was severe the problems concerned mental handicap and dependency. (See also Section IV on 'Educational attainments'.)

JENSEN, G.D.,
and KOGAN, K.L.
(1962)
*Journal of Mental
Deficiency
Research*, 6, 1,
56–64.

Parental estimates of the future achievement of children with cerebral palsy

110 parents (65 mothers and 45 fathers) of 68 cerebral palsied children, all under the age of six years and attending a spastic children's clinic and pre-school in Seattle, Washington, filled out a questionnaire designed to elicit their estimates of the child's future abilities. Compared with the average ratings of all the clinic staff, both mothers and fathers significantly overestimated their child's future skills. Only 12 of the parents underestimated the child. Children with severer mental or physical handicaps were more likely to be overestimated than the less handicapped, and younger children were more likely to be overrated than older children. Underestimation of the child by the parents or their failure to become more realistic as the child grows older may indicate disturbed parent–child relationships and suggest the need for counselling.

BARCLAY, A.
and VAUGHT, G.
(1964)
*American Journal
of Mental
Deficiency*, 69,
62–5.

Maternal estimates of future achievement in cerebral palsied children

Forty mothers of cerebral palsied children significantly overestimated, on average, their children's future educational, vocational and social achievements compared with the estimates of the investigators (based on standardized test scores). The extent of overestimation was not affected by the child's age or the severity of the physical handicap, but it was affected by his or her intelligence. The mentally retarded child was overestimated the most.

CARNEGIE
UNITED
KINGDOM TRUST
(1964)
Edinburgh: J. and
A. Constable
(Part I,
Appendices L and
M; Part II,
Chapters 2 and 3;
Part III, Chapter
5.)

Handicapped Children and their Families

Studies of children with cerebral palsy and their families were made as part of a larger survey of the needs of all types of handicapped children. Research was carried out in three areas, Glasgow, Sheffield and Shropshire. A mass of data on the practical problems involved in the care of cerebral palsied children was accumulated. Anxiety and strain occurred in a high proportion of the mothers. Few parents accepted the child's handicap. Only a small minority of siblings, though, appeared to be adversely affected by the cerebral palsied child's presence in the family.

SCHAFFER, H.R.
(1964)
*International
Journal of Social
Psychiatry*, 10, 4,
266–75.

The too-cohesive family: a form of group pathology

This study considers one possible effect of a stressful situation – the presence of a young cerebral palsied child – on 30 Scottish working-class families. The time spent together by the members of the families differed considerably, but 13 families in which the members were rarely apart, except when at work or school, were termed 'too-cohesive'. In these families all activities centred round the handicapped child and for both parents contacts with neighbours and friends and leisure pursuits were practically non-existent. Other siblings were not regarded by the parents in their own right but for the help they could give to the handicapped child, and sometimes the siblings themselves endorsed this position. The children in these families were no more severely handicapped, either physically or mentally, than those in the rest of the sample, nor were neighbours and relatives more hostile.

It is suggested that the excessive concern about handicapped children is due to the repression by the parents of their negative feelings about them. One indication of this was the inability of the parents to put even mild pressure on the children, so that they failed to encourage the development of self-help skills. The unity of these families is precarious, removal of the handicapped children for any reason being likely to cause disruption. The effect on the cerebral palsied children themselves was to make them socially immature, dependent emotionally on the parents and unable to cooperate with adults or children outside the family.

MORGENSTERN,
M.
(1966)
*Dissertation
Abstracts*, 26,
4079.

Maternal attitudes and reactions of normal siblings in families with a cerebral palsied child

The mother and one of the able-bodied siblings were administered psychological tests in two groups of 30 families, comparable in all selected criteria except that families in one group each had a cerebral palsied boy, aged between 5 and 17 years, as a member. Discrepancies in mothers' attitudes towards a cerebral palsied child and a normal sibling were significantly greater than discrepancies in attitude towards two normal children. Siblings of cerebral palsied children were more anxious and emotionally unstable than those with only normal siblings. The emotional reactions of the normal siblings were related to the mothers' attitudes.

ADAMS, M.E.
(1968)
*Cerebral Palsy
Journal*, 29, 2,
3–7.

Problems of management of mentally retarded children with cerebral palsy

A discussion of the psychological reactions occurring in families with a severely handicapped mentally retarded child at home. The child's very slow development may result in the parents becoming over-protective and failing to incorporate training in self-help skills into their care. Over-protective attitudes not only lead to dependence in the retarded child but also mean that the needs of the other siblings are neglected and a stressful situation created. Only practical help from the community, including clinical evaluation of the child, physical treatment, training outside or inside the home, and home help, can alleviate these problems.

KEITH, R.A. and
MARKIE, G.S.
(1969)
*Developmental
Medicine and
Child Neurology*,
11, 6, 735–42.

Parental and professional assessment of functioning in cerebral palsy

Previous studies have suggested that parents of children with cerebral palsy overestimate their abilities compared with the evaluation of professionals. In this study parents of 17 cerebral palsied nursery school children, as a group, rated their children more highly on current and future independent behaviour than did the school paediatrician, teacher, occupational therapist and physiotherapist. Parents' evaluations, though, varied widely, only ten of the parents actually making overestimations. Parents of children with lower Gesell Developmental Quotients tended to overestimate ability more than the parents of those with higher IQs, but age and severity of handicap did not have significant effects. The professionals also differed among themselves in their judgements. It is suggested that some optimism in the parents may help to sustain them.

BOBATH, B. and
FINNIE, N.R.
(1970)
*Developmental
Medicine and
Child Neurology*,
12, 5, 629–35.

Problems of communication between parents and staff in the treatment and management of children with cerebral palsy

From responses to a questionnaire given to 45 parents of children attending the Western Cerebral Palsy Centre, London, it was concluded that staff should avoid medical and technical terms in discussion with parents; that simple explanations should be given of cerebral palsy and the difficulties it produces for each child; that the instructions to parents should be given intelligibly and the close link between treatment and everyday activities emphasized; and that the parents should be kept informed of the child's progress during treatment.

HEWETT, S. WITH
NEWSOM, J.
and E.
(1970)
London: Allen
and Unwin
(Especially
Chapters 4, 5 and
9.)

The Family and the Handicapped Child

A study of the practical problems and effects on everyday life of looking after a cerebral palsied child at home. 180 mothers of children with cerebral palsy (aged one to eight years) from the East Midlands area were interviewed. 25 per cent of the cerebral palsied children were rated as being very mildly handicapped and 25 per cent as very severely handicapped, while the rest were moderately handicapped. 25 per cent of the children were of normal intelligence.

Child-rearing practices were very much the same as in the families with only normal children – although slightly more than half of the mothers did make allowances for the handicapped child. Jealousy of the handicapped child occurred no more often among the siblings than it did between brothers and sisters in families where all the children were normal. Only a minority (21 per cent) of the mothers felt socially isolated and the parents went out together as often as did those of normal four-year-olds. No judgements were made as to whether the parents 'accepted' the child's handicap, as the parents face a very complex situation and 'acceptance' is not necessarily a good or bad attitude. All topics discussed are illustrated with many quotations from the mothers.

MINDE, K.,
SILVER, S., and
KILLOU, D.
(1971)
Laval Médical,
42, 1041–8.

Some aspects of cerebral palsy and its treatment as perceived by the families of 49 children

The parents and teachers of 49 young children from a school for the handicapped in Montreal were interviewed about their experiences with the children. About half the children were retarded (IQ below 80) and their handicaps (mostly cerebral palsy) ranged from moderate to severe. Parents were asked about life circumstances, the child's history, the present status of the handicap, and plans for the future; teachers were asked to rate the children's emotional adjustment on the Rutter scale.

A quarter of parents knew of the handicap in the first year, a further 30 per cent in the second year, and the rest learned later still. Only half the parents felt they had received a good medical explanation, and only 30 per cent had a permanent and helpful doctor. 65 per cent wanted more discussion and information as well as practical help. The same proportion said that the child was aware of his or her difference from other children; a number stated that the children sometimes used the handicap successfully to get extra attention. The great majority said they had good friends and neighbours who accepted the handicap. Only three of the families had faced the fact that the future would be difficult for the child; the others stated that things would be all right or that they never thought of the future. Nevertheless nearly all estimated their child's mental ability accurately. The authors criticize the adequacy of the support given to parents of handicapped children, and recommend in particular that doctors should help them to face the long-term future.

McMICHAEL, J.K. (1971b) London: Staples Press.

Handicap. A Study of Physically Handicapped Children and their Families

A major emphasis of this study of 50 children (21 with cerebral palsy) attending a school for the physically handicapped in London was on the emotional adjustment of the children and their parents (see also Section II on 'Emotional and social adjustment'). The crucial factor in the children's adjustment appeared to be the degree and quality of the parents' anxiety and particularly the extent of parental rejection. 56 per cent of the parents were found to show moderately severe degrees of over-anxiety and failure to adjust. Factors which related to the parents' adjustment included fears about the child's future, anxieties about having further children, marital tensions, ill-health and the effects of social conditions. The major social problem in these families was housing, the majority living either in overcrowded houses with poor facilities or high up in blocks of flats.

SHERE, E.S. (1971) *Israel Annals of Psychiatry and Related Disciplines*, 9, 1, 52–9.

Modes of child-rearing in cerebral palsy: effects upon the child's psychological development

It is suggested that a young child with severe cerebral palsy, who can neither move towards objects nor ask for them, will be handicapped in that aspect of cognitive development which is concerned with the differentiation of objects and the exploration of their properties, unless the mother adequately provides the child with objects.

In the first two phases of this study, 13 mothers of young cerebral palsied children (mean age 3:7 years, mean mental age 1:4 years) were interviewed and observed in their normal activities with the child at home. The mothers were primarily concerned with the child's physical handicap, did not give toys or other objects for play and did not realize that a barren environment hinders a child's cognitive development. In the third, guidance, phase of the study, mothers were taught the principles of child development and supervised in play periods with the child. Most of them made some response to the ideas and some changes in their approach to the child.

KOGAN, K.L.,
TYLER, N., and
TURNER, P.
(1974)
*Developmental
Medicine and
Child Neurology,*
16, 4, 518–27.

The process of interpersonal adaptation between mothers and their cerebral palsied children

Ten cerebral palsied children aged one to four and their mothers were studied over a two-and-a-half-year period in the USA. The degree of handicap in the child ranged from mild to severe. Six 'interaction sessions' were recorded every ten months for each child: two sessions of play between mother and child, two of physical therapy conducted by the mother, and two of physical therapy conducted by the clinic therapist. The sessions were observed through a one-way mirror, and a tape recorder and video recorder were also used. Affection, involvement, and interaction were then each rated on a 7-point scale.

The authors found that positive and warm behaviour on the mother's part decreased considerably in both the therapy and the play sessions over the two-and-a-half years, and the same decrease was observed in the therapists. This decrease was clearly linked with lack of movement and progress in the child. The findings suggest that there is a gradual reduction in the amount of positive feeling expressed by those who work closely with these children, especially if they do not learn to walk. The authors argue that, since families typically invest much time and energy to the care of a handicapped child, they need professional reassurance that their efforts are valuable, and that the child who does not learn to walk may have other assets.

DROTAR, D.,
BASKIEWICZ, A.,
IRVIN, N.,
KENNELL, J., and
KLAUS, M.
(1975)
Pediatrics, 56, 5,
710–17.

The adaptation of parents to the birth of an infant with a congenital malformation: a hypothetical model

Interviews were held with parents of 20 children with a range of common congenital malformations hospitalized in Ohio. Timing of the interviews ranged from within a few days of birth to as long as five years later, 65 per cent being in the first year. Parents were asked a series of open-ended questions to determine their emotional reactions and perception of the child's handicap.

A number of common themes emerged, and five stages of reaction were delineated. Shock: the initial response was overwhelming shock. All but two parents reported a sense of abrupt disruption of normality. Denial: many tried to escape or deny the situation. Sadness, anger, anxiety: this accompanied and followed denial. Seven families reported feeling anger towards themselves, the baby, or hospital staff and others.

Eleven described intense feelings of anxiety. Five spontaneously spoke of fears that the baby might die and this seemed related to hesitance seen in almost all the mothers regarding their attachment to the child. Adaptation: ten reported a gradual lessening in anxiety and confidence in their ability to care for the child. Many mothers emphasized the child's normal qualities, and this appeared to reflect positive adaptation rather than denial of the disability. Reorganization: a complex time in which a more rewarding level of interaction with the child was described. Some parents continued to search for causes of the disability, while three seemed content that it had 'just happened'. Positive long-term acceptance involved parents' mutual support of one another, seven couples reporting that they had relied closely on one another, and six that the experience had brought them closer together. Asynchronous parental reactions often resulted in temporary emotional separation and may be a significant factor in separations following major family crises.

Marked loneliness and anxieties immediately after the birth were common, and the study suggests that generally the child should be brought to the parents as soon as possible after birth and the problems discussed, emphasizing the infant's normal attributes. Paediatric advice, support and counselling during the first year of the baby's life are crucial to maximizing the child's development and the adjustment of the family.

UNIVERSITY OF YORK, DEPARTMENT OF SOCIAL ADMINISTRATION AND SOCIAL WORK (1976)

Some Practical Consequences of Caring for Handicapped Children at Home

To gain insight into families' experience of available welfare services, interviews were held with 303 families with a severely handicapped child. Only 16.2 per cent of the families felt they had enough help with their tasks. 59 per cent said they only occasionally saw a health visitor and of those who were visited by one nearly half found the visits of no help. Three-quarters rarely saw a social worker. Of those who had had contact with the social services department, nearly a quarter had asked for practical help but been refused; the majority of their requests appeared to have been for things that had been provided for other families in other areas and at other times.

Of those with special equipment to help the child in the home, a third had bought it themselves, and in other cases the social services department had paid only part of the cost. Nearly three-quarters still needed other home aids. Where adaptation of the home to the handicapped child's needs were concerned, half the entire sample were unaware that social services could help with the cost; only 22.4 per cent had had an adaptation fully paid for. 63 per cent of the families felt that they still needed adaptations of various kinds.

Mobility equipment was needed for the child by 34.8 per cent of the families. Questions were also asked about the need for someone to relieve parents temporarily of the child's care; the majority did not want to send the child away, but alternatives in the form of home helps or child-minders were a possibility that would have been appreciated. In general, the study found a poor level of provision for the families of handicapped children, and there was a need for a single specialist worker to coordinate and advise.

LLOYD-
BOSTOCK, S.
(1976)
*Child: Care,
Health and
Development*, 2,
6, 325–38.

Parents' experiences of official help and guidance in caring for a mentally handicapped child

A sample of 97 parents of mentally handicapped children replied to a postal questionnaire asking, first, about the effects their child had on various aspects of family life, and, secondly, their experience of services provided. On the first question the general impression was that in spite of difficulties they loved and valued the handicapped child; nevertheless, stress, anxiety and tiredness were mentioned. Parents felt that the effects on siblings were generally positive, although jealousy and other problems occurred. Social life, family outings and holidays were greatly curtailed by the presence of the handicapped child, and this was more important than problems with housing or expenses.

On the question of provision of services, there was a great variation between regions. Many parents described long struggles for recognition and placement of the child, and learned to rely on themselves rather than to expect help. There were particular anxieties about facilities for older teenagers. Much depended on specifically helpful or unhelpful individuals. The most frequent suggestion for improvement was more specialist training for those responsible for the handicapped. For the majority of parents, obtaining help from services was more of a problem than the handicap itself.

BUTLER, N.,
GILL, R.,
POMEROY, D.,
and FEWTRELL,
J.
(1978)
Bristol:
Department of
Child Health,
University of
Bristol.

Handicapped Children: Their Homes and Life Styles

A detailed study of the life problems of the families of 255 handicapped children aged 7 to 17 in the county of Avon. 58 per cent of the children were mentally handicapped, 33 per cent physically handicapped (chiefly by cerebral palsy or spina bifida), and 9 per cent multiply handicapped both mentally and physically. Many findings are relevant to the care of children with cerebral palsy and spina bifida: inadequacies in housing, the problems of incontinence and broken nights, needs of wheelchair children, transport problems, depression and anxiety in mothers, siblings' problems, unawareness of available benefits. The authors report that many families were living in a state of constant crisis. If handicapped children are to be kept in the community, early and sustained support is needed for these families. The cost of putting the children into residential care is prohibitive in comparison.

BRESLAU, N.,
WEITZMAN, M.,
and
MESSENGER, K.
(1981)
Pediatrics, 67, 3,
344–53.

Psychologic functioning of siblings of disabled children

In 239 families in Ohio where there was a severely handicapped child with normal siblings (one-third of the handicapped had cerebral palsy), mothers completed a psychiatric screening inventory to assess the mental health of the sibling. The results were compared with data on a large sample of randomly selected children in Manhattan; it was found that the overall score for psychiatric disorder was no different for the two groups, thus disproving the idea that the siblings of handicapped children are necessarily likely to be maladjusted. However, on certain parts of the inventory, measuring 'fighting' and 'delinquency', the siblings of the handicapped children had higher scores than the other group. On 'isolation' they had lower scores. There was no significant difference related to the types of handicap or to its severity. Among female siblings, those older than the handicapped child were more at risk than those younger, while among male subjects those younger than the handicapped child were more at risk.

Section III: *Family Adjustment*

SIMEONSSON, R.J.
and MCHALE,
S.M.
(1981)
*Child: Care,
Health and
Development*, 7,
3, 153–171.

Review: Research on handicapped children: sibling relationships

A review of the research on sibling relationships within the family with a handicapped child. The discussion covers the influence of the handicapped child on siblings and vice versa, and the various factors that influence these relationships. The findings that emerge are contradictory and inconclusive; more sophisticated research is needed.

TARRAN, E.C.
(1981)
*Developmental
Medicine and
Child Neurology*,
23, 2, 173–82.

Parents' views of medical and social-work services for families with young cerebral-palsied children

A study of the problems faced by families of young cerebral palsied children in two Scottish cities, focusing especially on parents' feelings about services they had received for their children. The parents of 67 cerebral palsied children aged three to ten, with varying severity of handicap and attending two treatment centres, were given detailed interviews.

Nearly half were dissatisfied with the way they were first told of the child's condition, and more than half with the information they had been given since. Nearly half, again, felt they had been given no opportunity to discuss their feelings. Asked about the child's placement in a pre-school centre, half the mothers reported that they had been unhappy at first about the child being away for part of the day, but the majority of these soon found it made it easier to cope when he was at home. Most parents had found meetings with professional staff who worked with the child helpful. Asked who had helped them most to cope with the handicapped child, 28 out of the 67 named the doctor or assessment team, 19 named other professionals such as the health visitor, and 13 declared they had found no one to help. Two-thirds felt that having a trained person available for advice was important and in particular would have liked home visits. The author suggests that parents need early and continuing information, practical assistance with daily management, a home visitor, and contact with parents of other handicapped children.

COFFMAN, S.P.
(1983)
*Issues in
Comprehensive
Pediatric Nursing*,
6, 1, 67–77.

Parents' perceptions of needs for themselves and their children in a cerebral palsy clinic

Questionnaires were answered by 203 parents attending a cerebral palsy clinic with their children. The questionnaires listed subjects that parents or children might like to discuss with a nurse. 78 per cent of parents ticked off subjects they would like to discuss, and 34 per cent ticked off subjects that their children would like to discuss. Most frequent topics for discussion chosen were the nature of cerebral palsy, the child's development, and available services; least commonly specified were sleep, hygiene, and feeding.

GLENDINNING, C.
(1983)
London:
Routledge and
Kegan Paul.

Unshared Care

A study in depth of 17 families with severely handicapped children, some of them cerebral palsied. Long interviews about life with a handicapped child were carried out with parents, and their remarks are quoted extensively; the book gives a clear picture of day-to-day experience. The burden carried by the child's mother is conveyed, and the isolating effect of the situation. The overwhelming impression received by the author is that the families received far less help than they should; they were rarely made aware from the start of the various services available to them. Other problems were early difficulties in convincing doctors that the child was abnormal, difficulty in travelling and having any social life, and long waits at clinics without any facilities. Most parents gained a great deal of help from voluntary associations, but also contributed a great deal.

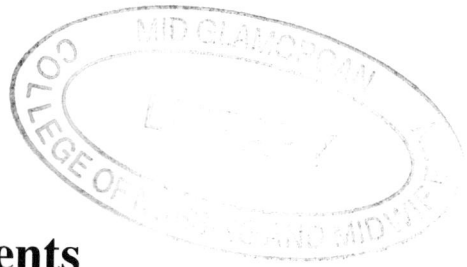

SECTION IV
Educational Attainments

Compared with non-handicapped children of the same age cerebral palsied children are, on average, backward in reading (Cockburn, 1961b; Barsch and Rudell, 1962; Rutter, Graham and Yule, 1970b; Yule and Rutter, 1970; Segal, 1971; Anderson, 1973) and in overall academic attainments (Cockburn, 1961b; Segal, 1971; Anderson, 1973). This is explained partly by the lower proportion of cerebral palsied children who have average intelligence or above (about one-fifth have IQs of 100 or above – Rutter, Graham and Yule, 1970b). Cockburn (1961b) found that attainments improved, compared with those of the average child, as intelligence increased and the severity of the physical handicap decreased (handicap tended to be, though by no means invariably was, more severe in the less intelligent). In one study of the school progress of cerebral palsied children (Bowley, 1967) it was found that about two-thirds of the children failing to make good progress were of poor intelligence and their reading and arithmetic attainments were mainly appropriate to their mental age.

Many factors, though, are involved in the educational backwardness of cerebral palsied children. Significantly more of the cerebral palsied children over the age of eight on the Isle of Wight, compared with the non-handicapped children, were retarded in reading by at least two years even when intelligence was taken into account (Rutter, Graham and Yule, 1970b). This could be partly, but not entirely, accounted for by the higher school absence rate of the cerebral palsied children. The authors suggest that direct effects of brain dysfunction – perceptual disorders and, of more importance at later stages of reading, language disorders – were partly responsible for the retardation (Yule and Rutter, 1970). A study of the cerebral palsied child's neuro-psychological deficits (Dorman et al., 1983) found that rhythm and pitch perception were closely correlated with reading and spelling skills; Gardner (1961) found that difficulties in spatial reasoning, maintaining attention and difficulties of social and emotional adjustment were the main causes of school failure in a group of hemiplegic children (mainly mildly handicapped). Bowley (1967) considered that limited speech, poor manual control and poor visuo-motor ability were the main factors in poor academic progress in her sample, in addition to lowered intelligence. Most athetoid children with involuntary eye movements which prevented focusing for any length of time failed to learn to read adequately, while children whose physical handicaps were as severe but who did not have eye movement difficulties learned to read (Pedder, 1964). While the severest physical and sensory handicaps tend to occur in those of lowest intelligence, even those cerebral palsied children with mild handicaps and good intelligence may be hampered by a wide variety of specific learning difficulties.

Nevertheless many children with cerebral palsy who have average or above intelligence are able to make good academic progress. In Bowley's (1967) study, 28 of the 41 children of average or higher intelligence were doing well at school, despite quite severe physical handicaps in some cases. Eleven of these children (mainly above average in intelligence) were at ordinary schools and all but three were making at least average progress. In contrast, in another study dealing with children at ordinary schools (Marlow *et al.,* 1968) only five out of the ten children studied were reading at the level expected for their mental age. The children were transferred to ordinary schools at the age of five or six years and the authors suggest that it would be better if such children remained at special schools, where their learning difficulties are better understood, until a satisfactory level in reading and writing is achieved.

Since this date a great deal more has been written about the possibility of integrating the less severely handicapped child into the ordinary school, both primary and secondary. Hegarty *et al.* (1981) in a survey of 17 integration programmes demonstrate some of the ways and means of achieving this, as do Hodgson *et al.* (1984). There has been little research actually comparing the progress and adjustment of handicapped children in ordinary and in special schools, but Cope and Anderson (1977), surveying special units attached to ordinary schools, found the children in the special units to be progressing at least as well as a comparison group in special schools.

Other types of studies summarized in this section include: follow-ups of the cerebral palsied after leaving school; investigations of intelligence distribution and stability in the cerebral palsied; studies of special groups of cerebral palsied, such as the deaf. The lack of research studies evaluating methods of teaching for cerebral palsied children with various problems is noticeable.

HOHMAN, L.B.
and FREEDHEIM,
D.K.
(1959)
*American Journal
of Physical
Medicine*, 38,
180–7.

A study of IQ evaluations on 370 cerebral palsied children

From re-examination of 370 children, it was concluded that 25 per cent of the sample varied by 10 points or more; least change occurred in the 50– and 90+ groups, and in children over six years. Variability in test results is about twice as large in cerebral palsied as in normal children, even though tests had been adapted to minimize motor handicaps.

COCKBURN, J.
(1961b)
In: HENDERSON,
J.L. (Ed)
*Cerebral Palsy in
Childhood and
Adolescence. A
Medical,
Psychological and
Social Study.*
Edinburgh and
London: E. and S.
Livingstone, pp.
281–324.
(Sections on
'Intelligence',
'Educational
attainment', 'The
implication of
intelligence and
attainment test
results' and
'Suitability of
existing
provision'.)

Psychological and educational aspects

Of the 223 children and young adults with cerebral palsy, living in eastern Scotland, only 26 had neither sufficient speech nor manual dexterity for intelligence testing, and these were all profoundly mentally retarded. Intelligence was found to average 67.7; about half of the cerebral palsied were mentally handicapped as compared with only 3 in 100 in the general population. There was a general tendency for IQ to fall as the severity of the physical handicap increased. Nevertheless there were a considerable number of cases where this relationship did not hold.

On standardized tests of reading, 73.2 per cent of the 153 cases aged over seven were able to make some score, but over two-thirds scored below the expected level for their mental ability. Only 24 children had reading or arithmetic attainments, or both, which were appropriate for their age. Over half the children could write legibly but one-third could not write at all. Writing ability was positively correlated with achievements in reading and arithmetic. Seventy school-age children were within the normal range of intelligence (IQ 70+), and without sensory handicaps, 43 being without serious speech, manipulative or motor handicaps and 41 of at least average intelligence (IQ 90+). Only 13 of the whole sample of 223 cases who were severely physically handicapped were not also mentally handicapped (and all but three were dull) so only very small numbers need special educational provision for the severely handicapped of normal intelligence.

The greatest area of unmet need found was in the provision for the 'ineducable' but 'trainable'. Forty-five of these cases were above school-leaving age. 53 per cent of them were assessed as employable. The majority of the unemployable were so assessed on grounds of mental handicap. Nine of those considered employable were not working, some for temporary reasons. Most of those working had unskilled jobs, sometimes involving long hours, and none were in professional or managerial types of work. Generally the provision for the cerebral palsied appears to become less satisfactory with increasing age.

GARDNER, L. (1961)
In: *Hemiplegic Cerebral Palsy in Children and Adults*. Little Club Clinic in Developmental Medicine no.4. London: Spastics Society in association with Heinemann, pp. 182–7.

Some educational and psychological problems associated with hemiplegia

Many hemiplegic children are mildly handicapped and can be educated in ordinary schools, or those for the physically handicapped. This study investigated 45 hemiplegic children who had failed in ordinary or PH schools. Difficulties could not be attributed to more severe physical handicaps or greater speech defects than in most hemiplegics. Although the children's average IQ of 60 was lower than that previously found in hemiplegics (average IQ 80), two-thirds were educable. The main difficulties appeared to be in spatial reasoning (30 per cent of sample), maintaining attention (50 per cent) and emotional and social adjustment (45 per cent). All these problems were more common among the left than the right hemiplegics. This suggests that the difficulties have an organic rather than psychogenic basis.

BARSCH, R.H. and RUDELL, B. (1962)
Cerebral Palsy Review, 23, 2, 3–10.

A study of reading development among 77 children with cerebral palsy

Reading development was evaluated in 77 children, aged 5 to 16 years, who were patients of the Cerebral Palsy Clinic in Milwaukee, US. 41 per cent of the children were attending regular (ordinary) schools, 34 per cent orthopaedic (for the physically handicapped) schools and most of the rest various types of special classes. There was no significant difference between the intelligence of those in the regular and those in the orthopaedic schools, the main selection criterion being the extent of motor involvement. 45 per cent of the children were judged as having sufficient intelligence (IQs of 90+ on clinical estimates) for learning to read successfully, but only 31 per cent of the total group were reading at or above their grade level.

Intelligence was directly related to reading ability in only 75 per cent of the sample, one-third of the retarded readers having average or above intelligence and one-fifth of the children with IQs below 90 being adequate readers. Failure to develop an adequate basic sight vocabulary and/or a system for attacking new words were significant factors in reading retardation. While lack of articulate speech may have been a contributory factor in a third of the group of retarded readers this did not appear to be of major importance for the group as a whole. The proportion of retarded readers was fairly similar in the regular and orthopaedic schools.

ABERCROMBIE, M.L.J.
(1964)
London: Spastics Society in association with Heinemann.

Perceptual and Visuo-motor Disorders in Cerebral Palsy

The cerebral palsied child is often handicapped in subtle ways in learning and comprehension, which only afflict children with neurological handicaps. Five chapters review the literature on these perceptual and visuo-motor disorders, and abstracts are included of 63 research papers.

GARDNER, L.
(1964)
In: *Learning Problems of the Cerebral Palsied.*
London: Spastics Society, 136–45.

The education of brain-injured children. A survey of 30 children with very uneven abilities

A study of 30 cerebral palsied children of near normal intelligence with visual-perceptual and visuo-motor disabilities. The children were those attending the Spastic Society's three schools for the intellectually normal who had a discrepancy of at least 20 IQ points between verbal and non-verbal intelligence test scores. Twenty of the children were mildly handicapped physically, and only three were severely handicapped, suggesting that perceptual difficulties are relatively independent of the severity of handicap. Reading ability at the secondary school level appeared to be similar to that of the other cerebral palsied children in the schools, but may have been somewhat retarded at the junior school stage. Arithmetic was more retarded than reading. On clinical judgements the sample children were more distractable, and possibly more emotionally and socially disturbed, than the other children. The author suggests that the setting-up of less distracting school environments should be considered for this type of child.

GARDNER, L. and JOHNSON, J.
(1964)
Developmental Medicine and Child Neurology,
6, 3, 250–60.

The long-term assessment and experimental education of retarded cerebral palsied children

A study of 41 cerebral palsied children of 'border-line educability' who spent a period (average ten months) at Hawksworth Hall, the Spastic Society's long-term assessment and experimental education centre. The children tended to have communication difficulties (51 per cent had severely limited speech, 22 per cent deafness which warranted a hearing aid and 17 per cent severe visual defects), physical handicaps which affected classroom work to a moderate or severe extent (cent) and emotional difficulties (45 per cent).

46 per cent of the children improved sufficiently over the assessment period to be up-graded to 'educable'. Improvements were made on various subtests of intelligence scales, in educational attainments, social-emotional development and 'drive and attention'. Differences between those found to be 'educable' and those who remained 'ineducable' did not appear to be attributable to the severity of the physical handicap, presence or absence of speech, home background or hearing loss. The 'ineducable' group, though, contained all the children with severe visual defects and more were firstborn (59 per cent against 21 per cent in the 'educable' group). The study shows that the 'ineducable' condition of the severely handicapped may be due to environmental factors and is not necessarily immutable.

INGRAM, T.T.S., JAMESON, S., ERRINGTON, J., and MITCHELL, R.G. (1964b) Clinics in Developmental Medicine no. 14. London: Spastics Society in association with Heinemann.

Living with Cerebral Palsy

A follow-up of 200 children and young adults, born between 1938 and 1947, originally included in surveys of the cerebral palsied in the eastern region of Scotland (Henderson, 1961 – see Cockburn (1961b)). At the time of follow-up, 43 of the cerebral palsied were in open employment (mainly unskilled), 32 in niche employment (allowances were made for the disability), five in sheltered employment and 14 in sheltered training. Eighty-eight were unemployed and 18 were still at school.

Chances of obtaining and keeping employment were better for males (47 per cent employed) than females (39 per cent employed). Subjects with hemiplegia found it easier to get work (48 per cent) than those with diplegia (33 per cent) or dyskinesia (20 per cent) because their physical handicaps were lighter. More of the mildly handicapped were in open or 'niche' employment (56 per cent) than the moderately (24 per cent) or severely handicapped (none).

Intelligence was also an important factor in ability to find work, for while 92 per cent of those with mild physical handicaps and IQ above 90 were employed, only 32 per cent with IQs below 70 obtained employment. Nevertheless some subjects with significant physical handicaps and mental retardation managed to obtain and keep work. Epilepsy, speech defects and unprepossessing appearance were factors adversely affecting employment chances. Those from the higher social classes and stable families had better chances of finding employment. Generally subjects who had attended ordinary schools obtained open or niche employment, exceptions being those with emotional disorders. (See also Section II on 'Emotional and social adjustment'.)

PEDDER, R.A.
(1964)
Spastics Quarterly, 13, 3, 20–7.

Reading skills of the cerebral palsied

The acquisition of reading skills was compared in three groups of six cerebral palsied children each. The groups were not 'matched' but they were as similar as possible in age, experiences, physical condition and intelligence. The first group (all spastic diplegics) had visuo-spatial and/or visuo-motor disorientation, but all achieved a reading age of nine plus years between the ages of 9:6 and 12:6. The second group (five out of six were athetoid quadriplegics) all had some degree of involuntary movements, including eye movements which prevented direct focusing for any length of time. Despite the greater physical involvement this group was far superior to the first group in copying geometric figures and drawing-a-man. Only one child reached the nine plus reading level during the period of study and he was 16 years old. The third group (all but one athetoid quadriplegics) had quite severe involuntary movements but did not have the same difficulty in eye movements as the second group. All the children reached the nine-year reading level between the ages of nine and 12.

ZIMMERMAN, I.L. and JONES, M. (1965)
Exceptional Children, 31, 9, 486.

Changes in intellectual ratings of cerebral palsied children with and without pre-nursery school training

Cerebral palsied children (age range eight months to 3½ years, average IQ 67.7, initially) gained significantly in social skills and general adaptability after six months' attendance at a pre-nursery school for cerebral palsied children. Intellectual changes were minimal, though, and the average change was not significantly different from that of a group of cerebral palsied children of similar age, intelligence and sex distribution, who did not attend a pre-nursery school.

KLAPPER, Z.S. and BIRCH, H. (1966)
Developmental Medicine and Child Neurology, 8, 6, 645–56.

The relation of childhood characteristics to outcome in young adults with cerebral palsy

A follow-up study of 89 cerebral palsied young adults living in New York, who had been evaluated as children 14 to 15 years earlier. Initial IQ and diagnostic category were both related to the level of functioning in adult life. Spastics, particularly monoplegics and hemiplegics, tended to be the most successful. None of the subjects with an initial IQ under 50 was employed. Twenty-six out of the 42 in the IQ group 75 to 110 were in open or competitive employment or training. Self-care status (highly correlated with IQ) was closely related to educational achievements, employability, economic independence and social participation. Despite their good self-care status (59 were physically independent) and educational achievements (34 were high school graduates and 15 went to college or business training school) there was a high rate of unemployment (39), economic dependence (only three were completely self-supporting) and social isolation (22 were social isolates and only 17 were socially active) in the group. (See also Klapper and Birch, 1967.)

MARGULEC, I.
(Ed)
(1966)
Jerusalem:
Jerusalem
Academic Press
Ltd. (Especially
Chapters 6 and 7.)

Cerebral Palsy in Adolescence and Adulthood. A rehabilitation study: medical, social, psychological and vocational aspects

Report of a national study in Israel in which the majority of the country's cerebral palsied adolescents and young adults (aged 14 to 35) underwent medical and social evaluation. Of the 586 subjects, 198 for whom rehabilitation was considered possible but who were not already working or studying, were given a vocational assessment, including psychological evaluation, over a period of about three months.

The average IQ (Wechsler) of this group was 68.9, with 53.1 per cent having IQs below 70 and only 8.6 per cent normal or above. Subjects born in Israel, Europe or America had higher IQs than those from Asian or African countries, possibly due to educational neglect or the unsuitability of the tests used. Personality evaluation (by means of projective tests, interview and observation) suggested that three-quarters of the group had a tendency towards dependence and that this was only moderately related to severity of handicap. About half had emotional problems and difficulties in social adaptation. The best adjustment was found in the area of work attitudes, but even here nearly 40 per cent had difficulties. The only significant difference between the personality traits of those born in different countries was that those from Asia and Africa had better emotional imbalance.

72 per cent of those assessed were recommended for further education, training or employment, including 44 per cent for sheltered employment. Help in placement was given, in cooperation with the Labour Exchange and local social welfare agencies. On follow-up, six months to 2½ years later, 76 per cent of the recommendations had been implemented. The study emphasized the need for thorough assessment of the cerebral palsied, for sheltered employment, and for a special placement service.

BOWLEY, A.H.
(1967)
*Developmental
Medicine and
Child Neurology,*
9, 2, 172–82.

A follow-up study of 64 children with cerebral palsy

A follow-up study of 64 children with cerebral palsy (diplegics, quadriplegics, hemiplegics and athetoids were in about equal numbers), aged 5 to 16 years with IQs over 50, who had attended the Cheyne Centre for Spastic Children for their nursery and infant education. Thirty-six were attending schools for the physically handicapped, 17 were in residential or hospital schools and 11 were at ordinary schools.

The 28 children who were making good progress were all of average intelligence or above, but they had quite severe handicaps, including epilepsy, vision, speech and hearing defects. Poor or absent speech was an important factor in the poor progress of 13 children who had good intelligence. In the 23 other children making poor progress the primary cause appeared to be poor intelligence – but speech defects, poor manual control and poor visual-motor ability were additional handicaps. All the children at ordinary schools were at least of average intelligence and none had severe physical defects. Only three of these 11 children were making below average progress and only three (including one making below average progress) showed signs of emotional distress. 45 per cent of all the children appeared to be well adjusted at school.

Social maturity was rated by parents in 30 cases (on the Vineland Social Maturity Scale) and was found to be similar to mental age in 18 children. In the 12 children who had a social age below mental age this appeared to be due to the severity of the handicap, parental over-protection or low intelligence. Most of the parents (52 of the 58 assessed) were judged to be 'realistic, constructive and affectionate' towards their children. Mothers' attitudes were probably influenced by the help and advice received from the Centre.

COTTON, E. and
PARNWELL, M.
(1967)
*Special
Education,* 56, 4,
7–11.

From Hungary: the Petö method

Report of work at Luton, using the Petö method of conductive education, developed in Hungary. The method, which unites treatment and education under a teacher-therapist, is not a substitute for normal education but a preparation for it. The experimental group consisted of nine severely physically handicapped athetoid children, aged 4 to 13 years, who had previously failed to respond to education. The authors found encouraging results after a year. Assessment by the Spastics Society after seven months showed no great improvement in intellectual level, but positive trends in ratings (for five children) on Gunzberg's Primary Progress Assessment Charts, which measure self-help, communication, socialization and general and fine motor control.

KLAPPER, Z.S. and BIRCH, H.G. (1967) *American Journal of Orthopsychiatry,* 37, 3, 540–6.

A fourteen-year follow-up study of cerebral palsy: intellectual change and stability

Fifty-four cerebral palsied young adults, living in New York, part of a larger group who had been studied in childhood, were reassessed after 14 years (see also Klapper and Birch, 1966). 32 per cent of the original group had IQs of 90 or above and 11 per cent had IQs below 50. IQ distribution and representation of diagnostic sub-groups were not significantly different in the follow-up group from those of the original population. The mean IQ of the group increased by 6.5 points on retest. IQ increases occurred mainly in the monoplegics and paraplegics. Stability was greatest for those whose initial IQ was below 50 and least for those with IQs between 75 and 89. Changes in the latter group were mainly in the direction of improvement. (Of 17 showing changes of 15 IQ points or more, 14 made gains.) Educational planning for the borderline normal should take into account their potential for intellectual growth.

MARLOW, E., THOMAS, M., and INNES, A. (1968) *Special Education,* 57, 1, 8–13.

Spastics in ordinary schools

The progress of ten spastic hemiplegic children with mild physical handicaps and average intelligence, who had been transferred to ordinary schools at the age of five or six after pre-school education, was assessed. Five of the children were reading at the level expected for their mental and chronological ages, but three of these children were making less satisfactory progress in other school subjects. Only half of the children were reasonably emotionally and socially adjusted to school life. A considerable amount of teasing related to the child's handicap occurred. Large classes and frequent staff changes made it difficult for the children to receive individual attention or for their specific learning difficulties to be understood. It is suggested that children who are likely to have difficulties in learning to read or write should not be transferred to ordinary schools until a satisfactory level has been reached in these subjects.

MUTHARD, J.E.
and
HUTCHISON, J.
(1968)
New York:
University of
Florida in
association with
United Cerebral
Palsy Association
Inc.

Cerebral Palsied College Students: Their Education and Employment

Report of a number of research projects dealing with the college and post-college experiences of cerebral palsied students. Subjects for the college study – 80 (of 158 eligible) cerebral palsied students from Midwest and Mid-Atlantic states of the US, who attended college at some time during the years 1957 to 1960 – were interviewed and given psychological tests. For the follow-up study 117 of the original 158 responded to a postal questionnaire sent out in 1966. For both studies, a comparison group of 78 non-handicapped students who attended college in the same years was used. A third of the cerebral palsied students were mildly, a third moderately and a third severely handicapped. Two-thirds had speech disorders.

Significant findings include: (1) While all the non-handicapped students graduated, only 71 per cent of the cerebral palsied did. (2) Although adaptations were made in the examination procedure for about two-thirds of the students, many were reluctant to use non-conventional methods to help in studying. (3) A very high proportion of former college students were employed (88 per cent) compared with the proportion usually found (20 to 30 per cent) among adults with cerebral palsy. (4) The cerebral palsied students generally had lower salaries and fewer were employed in professional or teaching jobs than the non-handicapped (45 per cent and 63 per cent respectively). (5) Students in jobs related to their education generally had better academic records than those whose jobs were less related to their education. They were also more satisfied with their jobs. Their college courses were usually more vocationally oriented than those employed in less educationally related jobs.

POLLOCK, G.A.
and STARK, G.
(1969)
*Developmental
Medicine and
Child Neurology,*
11, 1, 17–34.

Long-term results in the management of 67 children with cerebral palsy

A follow-up of 67 children who had been pupils at Westerlea School in Scotland, which provided treatment and education for educable children too severely handicapped physically to attend ordinary schools. Twenty-four were in open, token (i.e. allowances made for the handicap) or sheltered employment and an additional 16 (in training, still at school or unemployed) were almost certainly employable.

Physical handicap and mental retardation were the major causes of unemployability; severe and very severe physical handicap and an IQ under 70 were found only in the unemployable group. Additional handicaps, such as speech and visual defects, or unprepossessing appearance, occurred most often in the severely handicapped and did not affect their chances of employment. Where such handicaps occurred in the less severely handicapped they did affect their employment chances. Hemiplegics had the best employment prospects (83 per cent were in open employment), and dyskinetics the worst (36 per cent employed), in accordance with the tendency for hemiplegics to be mildly and dyskinetics severely handicapped. At follow-up only five of the sample were considered to be very severely handicapped, compared with 17 at the time of admission, suggesting that the school therapists had contributed to the employability of the group.

GARDNER, L.
(1970)
*Special
Education,* 59, 4,
11–14.

Assessment and outcome

It was found that an experienced assessment team could predict a cerebral palsied child's educational prospects with reasonable accuracy in 81 per cent of cases. The children were all those (203) who had been assessed by the Spastics Society between 1959 and 1961, when aged 4 to 11 years, for whom a definite educational outcome (at severely sub-normal, educational sub-normal or normal intellectual level) was predicted and for whom information could be obtained five years later. Disagreements between prediction and outcome were greatest for children with minimal physical handicaps and those with severe sensory or behavioural handicaps who did not fit easily into one of the established categories of schools for handicapped children. Disagreements arose from unavailability of the recommended type of schooling, errors in assessment or changes within the child. In conclusion the author urges the setting up of locally based educational assessment units in which there can be a close link between assessment and teaching.

LOVE, N.W.J.
(1970)
*Exceptional
Children,* 37, 4,
301–2.

The relative occurrence of secondary disabilities in children with cerebral palsy and other primary handicaps

Sixty-one primary school (ages 6 to 12) physically handicapped children were given medical, psychological and educational evaluations. 84 per cent of the children were found to have secondary disabilities which needed treatment or special attention. Cerebral palsied children, as compared with children having other physical handicaps, suffered significantly more from mental retardation (80 per cent of the cerebral palsied, compared with 52 per cent of the 'others' had IQs under 90), speech disabilities (83 per cent, compared with 32 per cent), and secondary problems in general (92 per cent, compared with 74 per cent).

RUTTER, M., GRAHAM, P. and YULE, W. (1970b) Clinics in Developmental Medicine no. 35/36. London: Spastics International Medical Publications in association with Heinemann, pp. 133–49 (Chapter 9).

A Neuropsychiatric Study in Childhood

In the survey of all school-age children with neuro-epileptic disorders on the Isle of Wight (see also Section II on 'Emotional and social adjustment') it was found that a third of the children with cerebral palsy attended ordinary schools. School placement varied with the type of cerebral palsy. Half of the hemiplegic children were in ordinary schools and none under the mental subnormality services, while all but one of the bilateral hemiplegics were under their care. A third of all the cerebral palsied children were mentally subnormal (IQs below 50/55), while a fifth were above average in intelligence (shortened version of Wechsler Intelligence Scale for Children).

Again, IQ distribution varied with the type of cerebral palsy, only one hemiplegic being mentally subnormal while all the bilateral hemiplegics had IQs of 50 or below. 41 per cent of the cerebral palsied children over eight years were at least two years retarded in reading (in relation to age and intelligence (Neale Analysis of Reading Ability)). This may be partly due to school absences, which were greater among the cerebral palsied children than among a control group (evidence relates to 9- to 12-year-olds – see Yule and Rutter (1970)). Other factors must be involved, though, as a similar rate of absence was found among the physically handicapped without brain disorders, but only half the amount of reading retardation. Abnormalities of brain function are probably partly responsible.

STONE, M.C. (1970) *Exceptional Children,* 36, 9, 674–7.

Behaviour shaping in a classroom for children with cerebral palsy

Behaviour shaping techniques (consistently rewarding correct responses and not rewarding inappropriate responses) were used over a period of one school year in a class consisting of seven cerebral palsied boys (aged seven to nine years, with mental ages two to four years lower), all of whom, except one, had only minimal physical involvement. The class became more orderly, inappropriate behaviour, such as running from the room or hitting other children, being reduced. The children increased in their ability to sit still, concentrate on a task and pay attention to a teacher. Their ability to learn new tasks also improved. After a time the original reward (cookies) became ineffective and had to be replaced by another (pennies to buy toys). Appropriate behaviour never became automatic and tended to disappear once the children left the classroom. The author concludes that behaviour shaping is useful in dealing with classroom behaviour problems but that it cannot be used as a substitute for the establishment of an effective relationship between the teacher and the children.

VERNON, M.
(1970)
*Exceptional
Children,* 36, 10,
743–51.

Clinical phenomenon of cerebral palsy and deafness

An investigation of all the children (69) with both cerebral palsy and deafness who were evaluated at or attended the California School for the Deaf, over a period of 12 years ending 1964. Almost a half of the children were of average intelligence, or above (compared with the 14 per cent found in most investigations of cerebral palsied children in general). Compared with the non-cerebral palsied deaf children, 87 per cent of the children with cerebral palsy were below average in academic achievements (based on teachers' assessments of 45 children) and two-thirds or more were poor in speech, speechreading and language. Hearing loss was less than in the rest of the school population and lowered IQ only partially accounted for the deficiency in communication skills. It is suggested that a large part of the deficiency is due to neuropathology and resulting aphasia.

Many of the children were multi-handicapped, over a half having visual defects and a third being emotionally disturbed. The good intelligence of about half of the deaf cerebral palsied children suggests that they can be educated reasonably well. Early diagnosis and treatment of hearing, visual and other problems can enable them to make a fuller use of their capacities. Education needs to be specifically designed for the cerebral palsied deaf as methods used with non-cerebral palsied deaf children are completely inappropriate.

WILSON, M.M.
(1970)
Department of
Education and
Science,
Education
Survey, 7.
London: HMSO.

Children with Cerebral Palsy

Report of a survey carried out from 1957 to 1966 on cerebral palsied children in 30 schools and units (15 for children with cerebral palsy only and 15 for all types of physical handicap). 343 children were included, all those who were nine years old or under at the beginning of the survey. Aspects discussed include: the most suitable type of school for cerebral palsied children; special educational problems due to spatial and sensory perception difficulties; and different approaches to physical treatment.

During the survey period, 27 children were found unsuitable for education in school (after a year's trial at least), 15 were transferred to schools for the educationally subnormal, 24 to ordinary schools and 14 to a grammar school for cerebral palsied children. Of the school-leavers in 1965 and 1966, only 31 went into open employment and 23 continued their education at a training college for the physically handicapped, technical college or grammar school. Most of the others were in sheltered workshops (12) or day work centres (20), homes for the physically handicapped (19) or were unemployed and living at home (20). Problems of the severely handicapped after leaving school are very great and earlier review of possible employment is necessary.

YULE, W. and
RUTTER, M.
(1970)
In: RUTTER, M.,
TIZARD, J., and
WHITMORE, K.
(Eds) *Education,
Health and
Behaviour.*
London:
Longmans,
pp. 297–308.

Educational aspects of physical disorder

In a survey of all 9- to 12-year-old children with handicapping conditions, living on the Isle of Wight, 48 children were found to have brain disorders. The average intelligence of the 34 testable children who were above the floor of the Wechsler Intelligence Scale for Children (21 with epilepsy and 13 with structural brain disorders) was well below that of the control group. On average, these children were two years backward in reading accuracy and comprehension (Neale Analysis of Reading Ability).

Over a quarter were retarded in reading at least 28 months (in relation to intelligence and age) compared with 5.4 per cent of the control group. This may partly have been due to a high rate of absence from school, the children with lesions above the brain stem being absent twice as often as the control children. This cannot be the entire explanation as children with physical handicaps not involving the brain had a similar rate of absences, but only half the amount of reading retardation (14.3 per cent). Poor reading attainments appear to be partly attributable to the direct effects of brain dysfunction – possibly language and perceptual disorders. (See also Rutter, Graham and Yule, 1970b.)

NIELSEN, H.H.
(1971)
*Developmental
Medicine and
Child Neurology,*
13, 707–20.

Psychological appraisal of children with cerebral palsy: a survey of 128 reassessed cases

Findings from this study suggest that cerebral palsied children show at least as much IQ stability as children without neurological disorders or mental defects. Subjects were 144 cerebral palsied children (80 per cent spastic and approximately equal numbers athetoid and ataxic) who attended a Copenhagen clinic and were reassessed at the average age of 7.9 years after an average interval of four years, mainly because of medical or psychological problems. 55 per cent of the sample varied ten IQ points or less between the two assessments and 78 per cent by 15 IQ points or less. Greatest IQ stability was found in the children whose initial IQ was below 50.

SEGAL, S.S. (1971) London: William Heinemann Medical Books.

From Care to Education

A survey of one special school for the physically handicapped, with the primary purpose of investigating the nature and extent of educational backwardness. In the three school years from 1966 to 1968 the five main handicaps, accounting for over 65 per cent of the school's population, were cerebral palsy (30 to 40 per cent), poliomyelitis, spina bifida, heart conditions and muscular dystrophy, a similar pattern to that found nationally at the time.

In July 1967 when a series of five standardized tests were given to all pupils over the age of seven years at the school, backwardness was found in basic subjects in 65 to 89 per cent of children both at primary and secondary level. Intelligence tests made on four age-groups of pupils showed that the school population was below average in intellectual ability, 65 per cent having IQs of 85 or below. The largest number of intellectually backward children was in the cerebral palsy group.

On the Frostig tests of visual perception, 74 per cent of the pupils were weak in at least two areas (out of five). The greater the number of areas in which children were weak the lower their scores tended to be on word recognition and arithmetic tests. Cerebral palsied children, compared with the other main groups of handicapped pupils, had the highest average of weaknesses.

61 per cent of the pupils were in the maladjusted/unsettled categories of the Bristol Social Adjustment Guide. The proportions of emotional disorder were not significantly different among the brain-damaged group and the group without brain damage. Although there was some relationship between emotional disorder and educational backwardness, between 40 and 71 per cent in the emotionally stable/quasi-stable group were also backward on one of the attainment tests. A third of the 32 pupils leaving the school between 1963 and 1966 were not placed in open employment, including seven of the ten with cerebral palsy. It is concluded that the school cannot aim at a normal pattern of education without doing a disservice to the majority of the pupils.

ANDERSON, E.M.
(1973)
London:
Methuen.

The Disabled Schoolchild

A study of the integration of physically handicapped children into primary schools; the cerebral palsied form the largest group of physically handicapped children attending ordinary schools. Seventy-four juniors, with matched non-handicapped control children, were studied, and also a group of 25 from infant schools. In the junior group, the cerebral palsied made up nearly a quarter. The sample was drawn from seven local education authorities in town and country.

School placement: Nearly half the parents of the handicapped children reported dissatisfaction with initial procedures for school placement; about 13 per cent of the juniors had been refused at first by schools, and many parents had had to put up a fight to get placement in a special school.

Social adjustment: This was assessed for all children by a sociometric test, and the handicapped children proved to be less popular than their able-bodied controls. The cerebral palsied children received the lowest rankings. According to parents' reports, about half the handicapped children were teased, but teachers only reported teasing in a much smaller number. The teasing was confined to urban schools.

Behaviour disorders: All children were assessed by the Rutter questionnaires; no difference was found between the handicapped group and the control group (but both groups had higher scores than normal children in Rutter's Isle of Wight study – see p.53). Children with neurological abnormalities, such as the cerebral palsied, had a higher rate of behaviour disorder than the other handicapped children. For all children, antisocial behaviour disorder was much commoner than neurotic disorder.

Social competence: The handicapped children had lower scores than the non-handicapped children; neurological abnormality, severer handicap and lower intelligence were associated with lower scores.

Intelligence: There was no significant difference between the control group and the children without neurological abnormality, but the group with neurological abnormality had lower scores. The same applied to arithmetic and reading scores.

The author concludes with a discussion of how to integrate physically handicapped children into ordinary schools, and a comparison with school integration in Scandinavia.

O'REILLY, D.E.
(1975)
*Developmental
Medicine and
Child Neurology,*
17, 2, 141–9.

Care of the cerebral palsied: outcome of the past and needs for the future

Records were kept of all patients (about 1700) attending a cerebral palsy clinic in St Louis, Missouri, over 27 years. The sex distribution was 56.6 per cent male, 43.4 per cent female. Spastics made up 61.4 per cent of the sample, athetoids 12.7 per cent, and there were a number of smaller groupings. Further study was made of a sub-sample of 336: of these, 28 per cent were mentally normal and self-sufficient, one-third retarded and helpless, and the rest in between; 23.8 per cent were in employment, of whom a high proportion were spastic; 17 per cent had died; 11 per cent were in institutions. One-third of patients had no formal schooling, 26 per cent went to ordinary schools, 37.6 per cent went to special schools. 14 per cent went on to higher education. The author points out that figures for employment and education had not changed much over the previous 20 years at the time of writing, and emphasizes the need for more workshops and sheltered environments.

COPE, C. and
ANDERSON, E.
(1977)
London:
University of
London Institute
of Education.

Special Units in Ordinary Schools

A survey of special classes or units for physically handicapped children attached to primary and secondary schools in England and Wales. It was carried out by letter, visits, and by a comparison of 55 children at special units with 55 in special schools. The children, matched for severity of handicap, were discussed with teachers and parents and were individually tested.

The children in the units were generally equal in basic educational attainments to those in special schools. Facilities such as ancillary helpers and material resources, however, were less good in the units than in the special schools, except in the two purpose-built units. At the secondary level in particular there was a shortage of physiotherapy and of arrangements for PE classes. Children in special units and special schools expressed themselves as equally happy in their school lives. A higher proportion of special school than of unit children were not chosen as friends by other children. On a scale of social competence, the unit children had a significantly higher self-direction score than the other group. On assessments of adjustment and behaviour, both groups were similar. At the secondary level handicapped children did not appear to be segregated or subjected to teasing.

The degree of classroom integration varied from school to school, the main barrier being limited ability in the handicapped pupil. At the secondary level there was more flexibility and more mixing. At both primary and secondary level, social integration was easier to achieve than academic integration. In general, there was a fair amount of integration, which was beneficial to the handicapped child; but more could have been achieved if it had been a major goal for the school. The best units offered as good an education as the special schools, together with the benefit of contact with non-handicapped peers.

The authors recommend a shift in policy, towards more special provision within the ordinary school, and add 46 detailed recommendations about implementation.

RICHMAN, L.C. and HARPER, D.G. (1978) *Journal of Abnormal Child Psychology*, 6, 1, 11–18.

School adjustment of children with observable disabilities

Three groups of children were examined: 39 mildly cerebral palsied children, 39 with cleft palate, and 39 matched children without handicap. All children were rated by teachers for behaviour on a standardized checklist, and another test was used to evaluate achievement. Results showed that both the handicapped groups were more inhibited and had lower educational achievement than the control group. The fact that the two handicapped groups had similar profiles suggests that it is the presence of disability rather than the type of disability which counts. Lower educational achievement may be partly the result of a poor self-image.

ALLSOP, J. (1980) *Journal of Research and Development in Education*, 13, 4, 37–44.

Mainstreaming physically handicapped students

A practical discussion of the details of integrating physically handicapped children into ordinary classes. Headteachers should try to get to know the children before admission; and for the teachers, in-service training sessions can be held to learn about various disabilities. In the classroom, there must be adequate room for crutches and wheelchairs, and somewhere for children to rest. Practical adaptations to chairs and desks are suggested. The handicapped child should be subject to the same discipline as the other children, but school work may need to be adapted or scaled down. The class can be helped to understand something about handicap before the child arrives. Factors influencing the decision that a child can be successfully integrated are discussed.

HEGARTY, S.,
POCKLINGTON,
K., and LUCAS,
D.
(1981)
Windsor:
NFER-Nelson.

Educating Pupils with Special Needs in the Ordinary School

A three-year study of educational integration in 14 LEAs in this country. There were 17 integration programmes, ranging from nursery up to school-leaving age. Staff were interviewed at length.

Initiation: Procedures for starting an integration programme are discussed – talks with headteacher, preparation of school staff, telling the parents of children already in the school (not widely practised), preparation of the pupils themselves (also not very common). Things were frequently found to go wrong with preparation – handicapped pupils arriving before physical adaptations had been done, school staff not properly informed, initial support not maintained.

Staffing: The majority of the schools had special centres attached. Teachers staffing them varied widely in experience and background. Their duties included teaching the handicapped pupils, monitoring progress and integration, administrative work, giving information to ordinary staff, training, contacting parents, support teaching. Ancillaries were used in all the programmes studied, and their roles ranged from giving physical help to helping with school work or physiotherapy. They were sometimes assigned to secondary schools, which could lead to difficulties with teachers. Of the ordinary teachers, only 36 out of 242 interviewed said they had a good knowledge of handicap; 43 said they had no knowledge at all. The great majority said that specialized knowledge of handicap was important in teaching children with special needs. Nearly 40 per cent said they had received insufficient information about the handicapped children they taught, often because of medical confidentiality.

Support from outside agencies such as educational psychologists and speech therapists was often insufficient. Asked about gains and losses from the integration programme, the main gain mentioned by teachers was the lack of social prejudice in the non-handicapped pupils. Losses included difficulties with timetabling and classroom allocation, discipline problems, and the question of incorporating the handicapped child into teaching geared to the majority. The roles of advisory teachers, educational psychologists, physiotherapists, doctors and speech therapists are discussed. Training: it appeared that many programmes are operating without appropriately trained staff, and there is much need for training. Pupils' needs were going unrecognized because of lack of awareness or competence on the part of staff.

The physical environment: Some of the needs to be taken into account are parking facilities, a level or ramped approach, wide doorways, lifts or internal ramps, suitable toilets, treatment room, fire escape routes, accessible play areas, meeting places and lunch rooms, staffroom for special centre, meeting room for parents. Costing issues are discussed in detail.

The curriculum: A number of the schools' adapted curricula are described. Factors influencing the allocation of handicapped pupils to various programmes are distinguished. Teachers indicated ways in which they modified their teaching approach – e.g. giving more individual attention, simplifying material. They reported many practical difficulties in teaching children with special needs: inability to give enough personal attention, uncertainty about the child's potential, discipline problems.

Preparation for adult life: Courses were given for school-leavers, both in relation to employment and to general life skills. Special attention was paid in many schools to keeping records of the handicapped pupils' progress.

Social interaction: This was easier for the younger handicapped children than the older. There are many examples of handicapped children only associating with the other handicapped. Positive steps need to be taken to improve social integration, but there was some ground for guarded optimism. In general, the handicapped pupils seemed more confident and mature than they would have been in special schools, but less so than the ordinary pupils. They made some progress in independence and lost some of their over-sensitivity. There was, however, a minority who were aggressive, bizarre or sexually precocious. Ordinary pupils, in general, accepted them, though not necessarily as fully-fledged members of the community. Teachers' attitudes were very positive; and parents without exception wanted ordinary schooling for the handicapped child. The main conclusion drawn from the study is that integrated education *is* possible, and to a far greater extent than is currently the practice.

GRESHAM, F.M.
(1982)
*Exceptional
Children*, 48, 5,
422–33.

Misguided mainstreaming: the case for social skills training with handicapped children

The author reviews some 40 studies (mainly of retarded or maladjusted children) which show that the handicapped child is not generally accepted by his or her peers in an integrated class. He argues that mainstreaming is not in itself helpful, but that it can be if the handicapped pupil is given social skills training. He discusses research on suitable curricula for social skills training.

DORMAN, C.,
HURLEY, A.D.,
and LAATSCH, L.
(1983)
*International
Journal of Clinical
Neuropsychology,*
6, 2, 142–4.

Prediction of spelling and reading performance in cerebral palsied adolescents using neuropsychological tests

An attempt to measure the neuropsychological deficits which handicap the cerebral palsied in reading and writing. Twenty-five severely cerebral palsied adolescents with an average IQ of 86 were chosen for study. A number of tests were administered measuring ten factors including visual–spatial orientation, tactile sensation, and rhythm and pitch perception. Most scores were significantly below average. The factor most closely correlated with reading and spelling skills was rhythm and pitch perception. Studies of dyslexics and of patients with head injuries have pointed to the same factor as being important for reading.

HODGSON, A.,
CLUNIES-ROSS,
L., and
HEGARTY, S.
(1984)
Windsor:
NFER-Nelson.

Learning Together

Seventy-six schools in 21 LEAs in England and Wales were visited by the authors in order to learn how they adapted to teaching handicapped pupils. Twenty-six of them were then chosen for closer study. Aspects of their work that were studied include pupil grouping, organization of supplementary teaching, timetabling, modification of the curriculum, staffing, in-service training, and classroom organization and practice.

O'HAGAN, F.J.,
SANDYS, E.J.,
and SWANSON,
W.I.
(1984)
*Child: Care,
Health and
Development,* 10,
1, 31–8.

Educational provision, parental expectation and physical disability

A report on the professional attention received by 24 physically handicapped children being educated in ordinary schools, and on the attitudes of their parents. The age range was 5 to 12 years, and they attended 17 different schools. All had been referred to the child guidance service at some time, for various reasons. Child guidance records were scrutinized, and parents were interviewed.

Among the 24 pupils, 40 intelligence tests had been given, 43 reading tests, and 36 other tests of various kinds. Forty-one reports had been made to the schools altogether, though nearly half the pupils had had no reports about them. Parents had received an average of 2.2 letters or reports and 1.8 visits from psychologists; only three families had received none. In addition, there were a further 183 items on file, many of which were administrative.

Of the parents, 62.5 regarded their contact with professional advisers as poor, and none regarded it as good. In terms of who had been most helpful to them, nearly a third could not name anyone, and the most popular choice was the physiotherapist, chosen by 21 per cent. Only one parent named the educational psychologist as most helpful. 67 per cent would have liked more help from outside agencies. Most parents were very involved in the choice of placing the child in an ordinary school and were very satisfied with teachers' attitudes and children's progress, though they thought that teachers should have more medical information. They wanted the children to progress to integrated secondary schooling if possible.

The finding that parents were satisfied with schooling is encouraging. But in view of the amount of specialized professional attention paid to the children, it is a matter for concern that few parents felt they had gained any help from it.

SECTION V
General

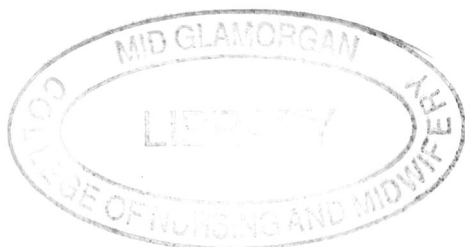

References are given in this section to a number of books and articles concerned with cerebral palsy not covered earlier in this booklet – aetiology, incidence, types of physical handicap, secondary handicaps, physical therapy and services. Also summarized are a number of works discussing the needs and problems of the cerebral palsied and their families.

YOUNIS, M.
(1966)
Chapter 10 in
HUNT, P. (Ed)
Stigma. London:
Geoffrey
Chapman, pp.
124–30.

The way I see things

Written by a spastic girl, this essay gives a picture of the difficulties and feelings of the handicapped.

FINNIE, N.R.
(1968)
London:
Heinemann.

Handling the Young Cerebral Palsied Child at Home

For parents, practical advice given in simple terms and aided by many illustrations.

BLENCOWE, S.M.
(1969)
Edinburgh:
E. and S.
Livingstone.

Cerebral Palsy and the Young Child

Written by members of the staff of the Centre for Spastic Children at Cheyne Walk, this book deals in non-technical terms with the physical and therapeutic aspects of cerebral palsy. Descriptions of the educational provisions for young cerebral palsied children at the Cheyne Walk Centre are included.

GARDNER, L.
(1969)
*Special
Education*, 58, 1,
27–30.

Planning for planned dependence

Ideas arising from a seminar, organized by the Spastics Society, are discussed. Follow-up surveys suggest that 50 to 85 per cent of cerebral palsied school-leavers will not obtain employment. For the severely handicapped an alternative life-style, involving social and leisure activities, needs to be planned.

WILLIAMS, I.A.
(1969)
Lancet, ii, 1126–9.

Management of the adolescent with cerebral palsy

Reassessment of the physical condition, intelligence and emotional stability of the cerebral palsied adolescent is necessary for planning his or her future.

Section V: *General*

DINNAGE, R.
(1970)
London:
Longman in
Association with
the National
Bureau for
Co-operation in
Child Care.

The Handicapped Child: Research Review, Vol I

Review of research on neurological disorders. A considerable part of the book is devoted to cerebral palsy. Twenty-five studies are abstracted and there is a comprehensive annotated bibliography.

YOUNGHUSBAND,
E., BIRCHALL,
D., DAVIE, R.,
and KELLMER
PRINGLE, M.L.
(Eds)
(1970)
London: National
Bureau for
Co-operation in
Child Care (now
National
Children's
Bureau).

Living with Handicap

The report of a working party of experts set up under the auspices of the National Children's Bureau to review the needs of handicapped children and the adequacy of the existing services for them. Evidence and information was obtained from professional and voluntary organizations, local authorities and from parents of handicapped children. On the basis of these contributions and their own experiences in various disciplines concerned with handicapped children, the working party made detailed recommendations on every aspect of their subject.

OSWIN, M.
(1971)
London: Allen
Lane.

The Empty Hours

A close study of the weekend life of mentally and physically handicapped children in institutions. Two residential schools for the handicapped are compared with two residential hospital wards, and the latter environments are shown to be grossly depriving and inadequate for the children living there. A serious indictment of institutional care for the handicapped child.

RICHARDSON,
S.S.
(1972)
*Developmental
Medicine and
Child Neurology*,
14, 4, 524–35.

People with cerebral palsy talk for themselves

A report of an informal discussion between three cerebral palsied people and the mother of a cerebral palsied teenager, held at a meeting for professional workers. Difficulties in relation to education, home and community life are discussed – the public's stereotype of the cerebral palsied, the problems of asking for help, the need to try out a non-segregated life. School work was felt to be interrupted too much by physical therapy. A need for sex education was expressed. Parents' attitudes are crucially important. The participants were dissatisfied with the way physiotherapy was carried out, and with doctors' understanding of cerebral palsy. In general, they stressed that they wanted to be treated as individuals rather than as cerebral palsy cases.

JACKSON, A.,
BURGH, A., and
WINSHIP, K.
(1973)
*Community
Medicine,* 129,
293–7.

The needs of handicapped children and their families in an East London borough

A description of the work of a hospital-based clinic for the comprehensive assessment and management of handicapped children (31 per cent cerebral palsied). Parents of the children were interviewed to find out what they felt their needs were. It was concluded that even more time and attention should be devoted to explanation of the child's handicap and future progress; much greater attention should be paid to the provision of equipment and its supervision; GPs should be encouraged to take a greater interest in young handicapped patients; more social support is needed for families of the handicapped; health visitors could give more help if they had more specific training; priority should be given to families with handicapped children for ground-floor accommodation; there is a need for nursery places for children too handicapped for ordinary nurseries; at least one residential home is needed in the district for short and long-term care; ultimately there should be a unified child health service within the proposed area health authority district, which could better meet the needs of handicapped children and their families.

MACKEITH, R.
(1973)
*Developmental
Medicine and
Child Neurology,*
15, 524–7.

The feelings and behaviour of parents of handicapped children

A brief resumé of family reactions to the birth of a handicapped child, from feelings of shock and bereavement at the outset to different types of parental behaviour – loving care for the child, over-protection, rejection, depression or adjustment. Professional workers faced with a handicapped child may experience the same range of reactions, and doctors' inappropriate behaviour may express a sense of inadequacy. Crisis periods during the child's life are also discussed, and the need for good support for the parents.

PILLING, D.
(1973)
London:
Longman in
association with
the National
Children's
Bureau.

The Handicapped Child: Volume III

Third in a series produced by the National Children's Bureau, this volume surveys in detail research on the mentally handicapped, both educationally subnormal and severely retarded, and thus is relevant to a proportion of the cerebral palsied. Over 300 books and articles published between 1958 and 1972 are listed, and all important studies are summarized at length. Aetiology, prevalence, care and education, assessment and training, family life are all reviewed and discussed.

FOX, A.M.
(1974)
London: Camden
and Islington
Area Health
Authority.

They get this training, but they don't really know how you feel

Nine taped interviews with parents of children with varying handicaps are given verbatim, and many issues important to them are raised.

LORING, J. and
BURN, G.
(1975)
London:
Routledge and
Kegan
Paul/Spastics
Society.

Integration of Handicapped Children in Society

Twenty-two contributions, taken from papers given at a study group sponsored by the Spastics Society and the International Cerebral Palsy Society, cover many different aspects of integrating the handicapped child into school and society.

CRUICKSHANK,
W.M. (Ed)
(1976)
Revised edition.
Syracuse:
Syracuse
University Press.

Cerebral Palsy; a Developmental Disability.

Written by recognized authorities in the field, this standard work covers medical, psychological and therapeutic points of view, as well as education and rehabilitation.

OUELETTE, A.E.
(1976)
*American
Archives of
Rehabilitation
Theory*, 24, 3,
52–5.

Cerebral palsy: the myth of a label

The author points out that in research projects and in society the person with cerebral palsy is judged by the disability rather than as a whole person with normal characteristics. At the end of therapy and education, society offers little except social isolation. The stereotype of physical perfection is reinforced by advertising, and the prevailing work ethic devalues anyone who cannot compete in employment. The author calls for a serious effort of re-education of public attitudes, in particular through group training sessions held for the disabled and non-disabled together.

BRITTON, E.
(1978)
Educational Research, 21, 1, 3–9.

Warnock and integration

In this article, based upon a paper read to the Annual Meeting of the British Association for the Advancement of Science, Sir Edward Britton discusses changing attitudes to handicap, challenges the medical model of the handicapped child, and distinguishes between handicap and disability. He examines arguments for and against the new hopes for teaching children together in an integrated setting wherever possible.

OSWIN, M.
(1978)
London: Bedford
Square Press.

Holes in the Welfare Net

For both ordinary readers and professionals, a readable and forceful account of some of the anomalies in the care of the handicapped which need to be put right – an account relevant to care of the cerebral palsied among others. The author describes how medical staff break the news of handicaps to parents; parents' search for information and advice; the specific problems of coping with handicap during childhood; special difficulties of adolescence; life in mental handicap hospitals and homes for the physically handicapped. In all these areas she finds a serious lack of sufficient care, and makes suggestions for improvements.

BOBATH, K.
(1980)
London: Spastics
International
Medical
Publications/
William
Heinemann
Medical Books.

A Neurophysiological Basis for the Treatment of Cerebral Palsy

Detailed discussion of the Bobath method of physical treatment.

BOWLEY, A.H.
and
GARDNER, L.
(1980)
In: *The
Handicapped
Child.
Educational and
Psychological
Guidance for the
Organically
Handicapped.*
Edinburgh:
Churchill
Livingstone, pp.
1–52.

The child with cerebral palsy

A comprehensive discussion of the educational and psychological aspects of cerebral palsy, written in non-technical terms for both the professional and the non-professional. Subjects covered include: psychological assessment; early treatment and training – physiotherapy, speech and occupational therapy and the radical and comprehensive approaches of the Petö and Doman-Delacato methods; early education; considerations in choosing the most suitable type of schooling for the cerebral palsied child; and the educational problems of the severely subnormal and intellectually gifted child.

RAPP, D.
(1980)
*Developmental
Medicine and
Child Neurology,*
22, 4, 448–53.

Drool control: long-term follow-up

Cerebral palsied children often have the additional antisocial handicap of drooling. This can influence placement even more than physical and mental handicap. At Meldreth Manor School for cerebral palsied children a small electronic behaviour modification device was constructed which provided repeated auditory cues to remind the child to swallow. The device was found to continue to be sucessful so long as the child wore the cueing device.

SPASTICS SOCIETY
(1980)
Parents'
Handbook No. 1.

The Early Years

Easy to understand explanations of diagnosis, treatment, care and management. Illustrated with photographs.

SPENCER, M.
(1980)
*Special
Education,* 7, 1,
18–20

Wheelchairs in a primary school

An account by the headteacher of a primary school taking in a large number of children with varied handicaps, and the adaptations and additions required for their needs.

TIZARD, J.
(1980)
*Journal of the
Royal College of
Physicians of
London*, 14, 2,
72–80.

Cerebral palsies: treatment and prevention

In the Croonian Lecture for 1978, the author outlines the history and diagnosis of cerebral palsy, and goes on to question the value of both treatment by physiotherapy and an insistence on early diagnosis. The question of prevention is discussed, and the present falling incidence of cerebral palsy.

COTTON, E.
(1981)
London: Spastics
Society.

Conductive Education and Cerebral Palsy

An introduction to the Petö method of physical therapy; six excerpts from articles and lectures.

DARNBOROUGH,
A. and KINRADE,
D.
(1981)
Cambridge:
Woodhead-
Faulkner in
association with
the Royal
Association for
Disability and
Rehabilitation

Directory for the Disabled

A resource directory of use to all concerned with handicap.

NEWSON, E. and
HIPGRAVE, T.
(1982)
Cambridge:
Cambridge
University Press.

Getting Through to Your Handicapped Child

Based on workshops with parents of handicapped children at the Child Development Research Unit at Nottingham University, the book describes in clear and simple language how to communicate with the handicapped child and structure his or her play, eating, toileting and talking by means of clear messages and rewards.

PHILP, M., and
DUCKWORTH, D.
(1982)
Windsor:
NFER-Nelson.

Children with Disabilities and their Families: a Review of Research

A survey of over 250 references, arranged under the following subject headings: the meaning of disablement; practical problems; parents' problems and adaptation; disabled children's emotional adjustment; siblings of the disabled child; information and services; voluntary organizations and self-help groups.

TITCHENER, J.
(1983)
Physiotherapy,
69, 8, 313–6.

A preliminary evaluation of conductive education

A description of seven months' use of the Petö method of physical education with eight cerebral palsied children in a special school. Preliminary results suggested some progress towards independence of movement and improvement in speech and self-help skills. The author points out, however, the lack of a control group, the problem of providing helpers for a 12-hour stretch, and the need to involve parents.

HARDY, J.
(1983)
Englewood Cliffs,
New Jersey:
Prentice-Hall Inc.

Cerebral Palsy

A book focusing specifically on communication disorder in cerebral palsy and its remediation; by the director of an American programme for speech therapy for the cerebral palsied.

SCHLEICHKORN,
J.
(1983)
Baltimore:
University Park
Press.

Coping with Cerebral Palsy: Answers to Questions Parents Often Ask

A useful book for parents, written with a minimum of jargon, and arranged in question-and-answer form. Some of the information about services and education are more relevant to the USA than to this country, but most of the subjects – types of cerebral palsy, causes, growth and development, psychological and social help – are of interest to British readers, and are covered thoroughly. A glossary of medical terms is appended, and a list of recommended reading.

THOMPSON,
G.H., RUBIN,
I.L., and BILENKER,
R.M. (Eds)
(1983)
London: Grune &
Stratton/
Academic Press.

Comprehensive Management of Cerebral Palsy

An up-to-date and detailed illustrated manual for professionals about all aspects of the management of cerebral palsy. Subjects covered include aetiology and prevention, assessment of associated dysfunctions, therapy and surgery, and social, educational and maturational considerations.

ROBINSON, A.
(1984)
London: National
Children's
Bureau.

Respite Care Services

A National Children's Bureau pamphlet which examines the role of temporary caring services for families with a handicapped child. Types of service available – residential care, family-based care, care in the child's home, holiday schemes – are described,

The Child with Cerebral Palsy

and the factors which contribute towards their success. Staff qualifications, both professional and voluntary, are discussed; research into the subject is reviewed. A list of names and addresses is appended.

ROBINSON, R.O. and McCARTHY, G.T. (1984) Chapter 6 in McCARTHY, G.T. (Ed) *The Physically Handicapped Child: An Interdisciplinary Approach to Management.* London: Faber.

Cerebral palsy

General approach; systems of treatment; types of cerebral palsies, their causes and management; drugs; training in independence; speech disorders; standing and walking; secondary structural deformity; education; emotional development.

SCRUTTON, D. (1984) Clinics in Developmental Medicine no. 90, Spastics International Medical Publications. Oxford: Blackwell.

Management of the Motor Disorders of Children with Cerebral Palsy

A number of leading practitioners discuss their views on treatment: the neuro-developmental treatment of the Bobaths, conductive education (Petö), the Portage Project model, aim-oriented management (Scrutton), Winthrop Phelps' Children's Rehabilitation Institute, Vaclav Vojta's treatment, sensory integrative therapy.

72

Author Index

Hewett, S. with Newsom, J. and E. (1970) 31
Hodgson, A., Clunies-Ross, L. and Hegarty, S. (1984) 60
Hohman, L.B. and Freedheim, D.K. (1959) 41

Ingram, T.T.S., Jameson, S., Errington, J. and Mitchell, R.G. (1964a) 13, (1964b) 44

Jackson,A., Burgh, A. and Winship, K. (1973) 66
Jensen,G.D. and Kogan, K.L. (1962) 28

Keith, R.A. and Markie, G.S. (1969) 30
Klapper, Z.S. and Birch, H. (1966) 45, (1967) 48
Kogan, K.L., Tyler, N. and Turner, P. (1974) 33

Lloyd-Bostock, S. (1976) 35
Loring, J. and Burn, G. (1975) 67
Love, N.W.J. (1970) 50

MacKeith, R. (1973) 66
McMichael, J.K. (1971a) 16, (1971b) 32
Madge, N. and Fassam, M. (1982) 22
Margalit, M. (1981) 20
Margulec, I. (Ed) (1966) 46
Marlow, E., Thomas, M. and Innes, A. (1968) 48
Miller, E.A. (1958) 12
Minde, K.K. (1978) 19
Minde, K.K., Hackett, J.D., Killou, D. and Silver, S. (1972) 17
Minde, K.K., Silver, S. and Killou, D. (1971) 31
Morgenstern, M. (1966) 29
Muthard, J.E. (1965) 13
Muthard, J.E. and Hutchison, J. (1968) 49

Newson, E. and Hipgrabe, T. (1982) 70
Nielson, H.H. (1966) 14, (1971) 53

O'Hagan, F.J., Sandys, E.J. and Swanson, W.I. (1984) 60
O'Moore, M. (1980) 5
O'Reilly,D.E. (1975) 56
Oswin, M. (1967) 15, (1971) 65, (1978) 68
Ouelette, A.E. (1976) 67

Pedder, R.A. (1964) 45
Philp, M. and Duckworth,D. (1982) 70
Pilling, D. (1973) 67
Podeanu-Czehofsky, I. (1975) 18
Pollock, G.A. and Stark, G. (1969) 49

Rapier, J., Adelson, R.,Carey, R. and Croke, K. (1972) 4
Rappe,D. (1980) 69
Richardson, S.S. (1972) 65
Richman, L.C. and Harper, D.G. (1978) 57
Robinson, A. (1984) 71
Robinson, R.O. and McCarthy, G.T. (1984) 72
Rosenbaum, P.L. and Armstrong, R.W. (1984) 6
Rutter, M., Graham, P. and Yule, W. (1970a) 15, (1970b) 51

Sanua, V. (1970) 3
Schaffer, H.R. (1964) 29
Schleichkorn, J. (1983) 71
Scrutton, D. (1984) 72
Segal, S.S. (1971) 54
Seidel, U.P., Chadwick, O.F.D. and Rutter, M. (1975) 18
Shears, L.M. and Jensema, C.J. (1969) 2
Shere, E.S. (1971) 32
Simeonsson, R.J. and McHale, S.S. (1981) 37
Small, J.G. (1962) 12
Spastics Society (1980) 69
Spencer, M. (1980) 69
Stone, M.C. (1970) 51

Tarran, E.C. (1981) 37